# The Legendary Bulldog

## Gabriel Michaels

The Legendary Bulldog
© 2006 Gabriel Michaels. All rights reserved.

This book is a work of fiction. Names, characters, settings and incidents are either the product of the author's imagination or used fictitiously. Any resemblance to actual events, settings or persons, living or dead, is entirely coincidental.

Printed in the United States of America

Published by BookShelf Press, Livermore, CA
www.bookshelfpress.com

The BookShelf name, logo and colophon are
the trademarks of WingSpan Publishing.

EAN 978-1-59594-032-2
ISBN 1-59594-032-4

First edition 2006

Library of Congress Control Number 2006921372

My deepest thanks with much love to:

God Almighty - for everything, especially Your mercy and grace.
Holly - my wife and best friend, for your love, support and hard work.
Jeff Cooper - my good friend, and great teacher who helped edit.
Ms. Randi Dubnick - my editor at Ampersand Enterprises. I am glad I hired you as my editor.
Ed Covolo - for your old style misspellings on the one that got away.
Marianne Kelly - for your awesome artwork.
Ami Shishani – for your wonderful artwork on the front cover.
Donna - my sister, for your input.

My Bulldog family members, past and present, because you and your ancestors inspired me to write The Legendary Bulldog.

## Clause, in laws disabling best friend to defend!

Land of the free, nice to sing this song sincerely rather than jokingly, which may soon be. For man's best friend, most capable to defend bloodlines may be at an end.

For ignorant politicians, wannabe dictators in their positions, plot, destroying dogs like a Rot.

All should rightfully have a fit, when one is attacked by a pit.

But dog fighters don't give a sh-t if you illegalize their canines, which they criminalize. For they shall still fight underground, where ignorant politicians aren't around.

Just like if you illegalize the handgun, thieves would laugh, having even more fun.

The respectable, responsible shall suffer, in seeing the seed of their favorite breed which has protected thousands in time of need for so long be gone.

The American Bull, to illegalize should be unthinkable, brought by the early settlers; they gave their lives protecting against meddlers.

The Mastiff, been around for thousands of years, to stiff this breed would influence millions of tears.

Let us think of a solution, in line with our constitution.

Perhaps harsher leash laws, especially on dogs with powerful jaws, and more hard time for dog fighters who commit this hideous crime.

Maybe a good citizen's test; let the human aggressive be put to rest.

Land of the free, politicians in high positions should uphold this sincerely.

For if put to an end, man's powerful protecting best friend.

You will have lied if you say you honor the ones who died!

Let this truly be land of the free and continue singing this song with dignity!

# CHAPTER I
# HOUNDS OF HELL

Early in the thirteenth century, in the town of Stamford, England, lived a wealthy man named Lord Albert Hutchins. He was slender with long, dark brown hair. Lord Albert had heavy bags under his eyes due to sleepless nights spent mourning the death of his beloved wife, who had died giving birth to his daughter, Helen, their only child.

Lord Albert's whole world revolved around his beautiful blue eyed, ash blonde, freckled-faced daughter. Whatever Helen wanted, Helen received, which turned her into a spoiled brat. At just nine years of age, Helen saw Amanda Fowler, a very dramatic "gothic" looking girl. With keen interest, Helen watched Amanda happily playing with her nine week old Mastiff puppy. For Helen, it was puppy fever at first sight.

Helen tugged on her father's coat. "Goodly father, I do wish to possess that young hound which doth lie in the arms of yon raven haired maiden."

Lord Albert stroked his beard, looked at his daughter, and saw her pointing at Amanda. "Art thou certain?" Lord Albert hesitantly asked, noticing the huge smile on Amanda's face and the wiggling tail of the pup.

"Quite certain," answered Helen.

Lord Albert, looking away from Amanda in shame, approached her father, a fat, greedy, man who was halfway to being baldheaded. Lord Albert handed Mr. Fowler fourteen-shillings. Within seconds, Amanda had her puppy taken out of her arms by her father, only to watch it be placed in Helen's arms.

Amanda's ghostly white face suddenly turned red with rage. "Fret not precious," her father told her, handing Amanda seven shillings. "Now daughter, thou hast money enough to buy thirty pups."

"I do not want thirty pups! Or any bloody money!" Amanda yelled, throwing the shillings at her father's feet in rage. "I only desire my own pup, which thou hast given me last week -- for my tenth birthday!" Amanda closed and opened her eyes, while inhaling and exhaling a massive breath. Facing Helen and Lord Albert, Amanda drew an imaginary rectangle in the air with her finger as she warned.

*"May a scarred curse, like that of my heart,*
*be bestowed upon thee, if ye neglect me beloved puppy."*

After saying this, Amanda burst into tears and fled. Lord Albert and Helen felt strong powers of darkness released by Amanda's words. Though only ten, Amanda already had knowledge of witchcraft. Her mother was a witch who had taught Amanda how to cast a spell. Amanda's father, trembling

1

and fearful that his daughter might turn on him, picked up the money before running after her.

Helen, making light of the matter, said. "Dread not father; I shall never neglect my pup!"

"I do hope not," her father replied, as he walked away with his hand on his beloved daughter's shoulder.

That day, Helen enjoyed her new puppy very much, so much, in fact, that she demanded another one the next day. Of course, she received another puppy that day. This went on every day for the next several months. At first Helen would hug, play with, and care for each new puppy like a mother tending to her baby. However, as the puppies grew older, she neglected them. For Helen focused all her attention on the newer puppies. Noticing this, Lord Albert would periodically try to reason with her: "Pumpkin, thou hast acquired too many dogs." He even would occasionally refuse to provide her with any more puppies. But upon hearing this refusal, Helen would scream and cry.

"I do love pups; they bring happiness to me. I must always have many pups to care for, unless thou dost not care for me. Thou must not love me any more, father!" Helen would scream and cry for hours. Her father's heart, breaking at each angry word, would always cause him to give in. To avoid having hundreds of dogs living on their estate, Lord Albert would take several of the neglected older pups deep into the forest, abandoning them to fend for themselves. On the way home, Lord Albert would stop to buy another puppy or two. Helen had so many puppies that she never noticed the ones that disappeared.

But the townspeople did take notice. The local hunters noticed that the cherished prey that had been abundant in the forest for so long had become scarce. Several of the townspeople tried to reason with Lord Albert. They pleaded with him to stop purchasing pups, not wishing for any more dogs to be abandoned in the forest. Lord Albert, however, would not hear of it. The good-hearted breeders refused to sell any more puppies to Lord Albert at any price. Unfortunately, there were breeders who cared more for money than dogs. These unscrupulous breeders learned that they could demand five times the normal price, and Lord Albert would always pay in an attempt to fulfill his only child's every desire.

Years passed. Helen remained a spoiled brat, unable to make any friends, and cared only for the new puppies her father continued to bring home. Well, she also enjoyed eating sweets, so much so, in fact, that she was the plumpest youth in Stamford.

One night Lord Albert drove his carriage deep into the forest, as he had done on so many other nights. He brought with him twelve of the neglected young dogs, taking them to where he had dropped off several hundred dogs before. However, this dry, cold night would prove to be different. On this night, at first Lord Albert thought he was hearing the souls of the abandoned dogs crying out. It sounded as though hundreds of the once beloved dogs were howling and moaning their heartbreak at the full moon. Hearing this, Lord Albert abruptly halted his horses, jumped down from his carriage and unloaded the twelve young dogs. For the first time, Lord Albert felt the guilt of having abandoned hundreds of young dogs in the forest. As he climbed back into the carriage, he felt a chill come over him.

As Lord Albert started to drive off, he held his torch to his right hand side. There he saw several hungry dogs close at hand. Howling and snarling with bared fangs, the dogs paced alongside his horses. Lord Albert slowly turned to his left hand side, only to see a similar sight. Lord Albert swallowed hard and shook with fear. In his panic, he dropped his torch inside the carriage. He quickly picked up the torch, but did not notice the spark that remained. Lord Albert threw his torch at the dogs. A fire quickly took hold in the forest, igniting first the underbrush, then the trees. The forest soon became an inferno. Whipping his horses furiously, Lord Albert fled in his carriage as fast as his horses would take him. The dogs pursued, biting at the heels of the galloping horses as they sped away from the burning inferno and towards the town. As they approached the Hutchins mansion, the more brazen dogs jumped into the carriage, knocking Lord Albert out and on to the ground. A few dogs stayed on and rode in the carriage, while others chased the horses. Several dogs attacked Lord Albert, whom they all seemed to remember. It was as if the dogs wanted to make sure that Lord Albert would never again abandon their kind deep in the woods.

Helen heard her father's cries and quickly ran from the mansion to his side. Seeing the dogs, she yelled at them to stop, crying out, "Leave my father alone!"

The dogs remembered Helen's voice and stopped instantly. They turned and looked at her with their drawn, half-starved faces. Helen slowly began to recognize a few of the dogs when she saw their eyes. It was as though both the dogs and Helen were simultaneously transported in memory to their earlier and happier times together. Their few short weeks playing together and feeling loved emerged from their collective consciousness. Helen could see the recognition in the eyes of the dogs, and she knew that they still loved her unconditionally. However, the dog's faces and eyes were not happy as she had remembered them. The faces were now sad and haggard, with droopy eyes that showed the pain of separation from their first caretaker. Seeing Helen again brought a fresh pang of separation. The dogs, howling as if their hearts had been shattered, turned and ran back through town, catching up with the rest of their pack.

The whole town of Stamford awoke to loud howling and what sounded like the stampede of bulls. As the townspeople peered out through their shutters, they saw a huge forest fire in the distance and hundreds of dogs running into town. The dogs were still chasing the carriage, although the townspeople were unable to see the horses hidden in the smoke and cloud of dust. For that matter, the townspeople could not tell it was a carriage, as it was now completely ablaze. No one was able to discern that this was a carriage on fire. What the town of Stamford saw through their shutters that night was a fireball of flame, with a few dogs that appeared to be flying on top of the flame. Through the dust and smoke, those closest to the fiery procession could not see the horses as they ran by, but only a glimpse of the, fast, agile dogs that managed latching onto the sides of the galloping horses. The illusion that this provided led the townspeople to assume that these dogs were ghosts that had ascended from the pits of hell.

As soon as the horses ran out of town, their reins caught fire, disintegrating in the flames, and allowing the horses to separate from the fiery carriage. The horses were powerful stallions. Their strength and speed enabled them to shake off the dogs and run to safety. Luckily for the dogs, the horses had led them near a herd of small wild pigs. The dogs found the pigs to be an easier meal than the horses.

Lord Albert had been bitten, bruised, and battered. The worst injury was a large bite on his face, which would leave him with a permanent scar. Helen held her father and cried tears of relief that he was alive. She also cried tears of remorse, for deep down inside she knew it was her fault that those abandoned dogs had turned vicious. Helen knew that it was her neglect that had led to their abandonment. It was her love that had broken their hearts. For the first time in her life, Helen realized what it would be like to live without the one person who, like the heartbroken dogs, loved her unconditionally. Recognizing her selfish ways, Helen apologized to her father through her tears. Her father, also crying, held Helen. Lord Albert tried to console Helen, accepting the blame for indulging Helen's selfish irrational demands.

"The fault is not thine that thou art thus. The responsibility is mine. I do love thee more than life itself! I did think that nothing should be denied my pumpkin. I was unable ever to ever tell thee nay, and thus 'tis I who have created the events of this dark night," he cried.

Helen shook her head to say no. "Father, do not blame yourself. 'Tis not your fault that I have taken advantage of your kind heart by making such unreasonable demands. I did learn at an early age how much you do love me and how hard it was for you to deny me my wishes. This night of terror, the pain you do feel, is all because of my childish behavior. Never again shall I abuse your love. Nor do I want any more pups." Helen paused, wiping a tear, before continuing, "especially after seeing the sad faces of those heartbroken dogs. For the first time I do see my own selfish ways. I now do know my responsibility. I am going to be very kind to the dogs that I now own. They shall all be loved for the rest of their lives. None of them shall ever be abandoned." Tears poured down Helen's face like rain as she thought about the poor dogs she had seen that night.

The next day, rumors began to spread over England about the dogs of Stamford. It was made known that this wealthy lord had abandoned hundreds of young dogs deep in the forest and had left them to starve. People spoke of the souls of those dogs that came riding through the town of Stamford on a cloud of fire under the full moon. The stories included the disfigurement of Lord Albert, left with a gruesomely scarred face. The storytellers warned the listeners to never mistreat mankind's best friends, the faithful and loyal dogs.

In the town of Stamford, the townspeople believed that the souls of the abandoned dogs would not return because Lord Albert had heeded the dogs' warning and had stopped abandoning any more dogs. However, every now and then on a full moon, it is rumored that the old dogs' souls still howl in pain. These dogs were given the famous nicknames, "Dogs of Doom" and "Hounds of Hell". Several families even moved out of Stamford because they believed if the Hounds of Hell returned, they would not be as merciful as before, but would kill and destroy the entire town. The forest where Lord Albert had abandoned the dogs was considered a very haunted place. No one set foot there for several years to come.

# CHAPTER II
# THE LEGENDARY EARL

A famous Earl named William Warne, but referred to simply as the Earl, who was tall, strong and handsome, with dark sideburns, was intrigued when he heard this story. The Earl had heard the story from many different people, and was astonished that each storyteller presented the exact same story. The Earl was unable to detect any indications that the stories were fabricated or even grossly exaggerated. The Earl decided to take a trip to Stamford and investigate for himself. There, he met Lord Albert and saw the scar on his face. The Earl tried to discuss the night when Lord Albert was attacked, but Lord Albert refused to discuss the incident. He felt responsible for the huge forest fire, and for the wild dogs running through town that night. Lord Albert was afraid that the townspeople would hold him financially responsible for the events of that night. Therefore, he refused to talk with the Earl and walked away.

The Earl had owned dogs all his life. He recognized that Lord Albert had been scarred by a very powerful dog of the Mastiff type. During his visit to Stamford, the Earl stayed up late every night waiting and hoping for the "Dogs of Doom" to return. He even used a large fishing net to make a dog trap that was to be used by being dropped on the top of the Dogs of Doom. He watched and waited. Finally, on his forty-fourth night in Stamford, which was a misty, foggy night with a full moon, his long wait was over. The Earl had closed his eyes and was dozing off when he heard a faint howl coming from far away. The Earl instantly opened his eyes, threw off his blanket and sat up. His eyes moved from side to side as he listened intently for more distant howls. A few seconds later, he heard more howling, this time even closer. The Earl put on his sandals, grabbed his dog trap and headed out the door. The dogs were now pretty close. Along with the sound of the dogs, he heard very loud footsteps, which sounded like someone running fast and hard. Soon, through the fog, the Earl saw horns, and seconds later a gigantic bull was visible, bigger than any bull he has ever seen.

In fact, the bull had just happened to escape from a local cattle breeder and had run into the forest close to the place where the abandoned dogs lived. The dogs tried to attack the bull while it was running, and this is what lured ten dogs into town, five small and five huge dogs. The dogs were either really huge or really small because very small and very large dogs had a better chance of surviving in the forest than did dogs of medium size. The small dogs had the advantage of speed like fast cats, enabling them to catch small rodents. The huge dogs had the advantage of enough power and size to take down bigger prey, like wild boar, which lived in the forest. The medium sized dogs were too slow to kill rodents, and too small to kill large prey, and unfortunately for them, there was not enough food out there for either the smaller dogs or the larger dogs to share with them. Therefore, the medium sized dogs would soon die. The ten dogs that the Earl saw were all very thin, all with their ribs showing, and looking like they had not eaten anything in three weeks. The five small dogs bit into the bull and tried to hang on while the bull was running. The bull, however, was much too powerful for the small half-starved dogs. He violently shook them off, sending all flying against a wall. The bull started to out run the dogs, and it looked like he was going to get away from them. Then suddenly, out of nowhere, a small, heavily wrinkled dog with a short snout, looking like a freak of nature, with god speed ran past all the other dogs. He came within two feet of the bull before springing into the air, biting the bull on the neck. Furiously, the bull began shaking his neck, trying to shake off the small dog. Wisely, the dog released his bite, then ran in front of the bull down a narrow alley, which came to a dead end at a brick wall. The dog's plan was to make the bull angry enough to focus only on him (which worked; in fact, the dog now had the bull's undivided attention) so that the bigger dogs could attack the bull more easily. Enraged, the bull chased the dog down the alley. The bull was just inches behind the dog the whole way. When they came to the end of the alley, the small dog with the short snout jumped against the brick wall, springing off of it with all fours, doing a perfect back flip over the top of the bull, and landing on the bull's back. Immediately the dog bounced off with all fours, landing safely on the ground, and managing somehow to miss the sharp horns by inches. The bull was so completely focused on the dog that he failed to notice the brick wall in front of him until the last second. Locking his legs in desperation, the bull tried to stop short, but failed, and smacked into the brick wall face first. The powerful impact cracked the wall as the bull dropped to his stomach, momentarily unconscious. The bigger dogs caught up with the bull and attacked as a pack just as the powerful animal came to. Filled with rage, the bull rose to his feet, swinging his neck around. The right horn hooked one of the large dogs right in the throat. With all of his strength, the bull lifted his head in the air, violently shaking back and forth. Eventually, the dog's head was torn off completely. Blood gushed out of the big dog's body, spilling all over the place. The dogs all froze at this spectacle, especially the small dog with the short snout and wrinkled face, for the dog that just had his head torn off was his best friend. Looking on with great sorrow at his best friend's head without a body, the small dog with the wrinkled face reminisced about the past. Three years earlier when he was a puppy, Lord Albert dropped him off in the cold forest to fend for himself. Within seconds, a medium sized dog approached, and being neither fast enough to catch rabbits nor strong enough to kill wild pigs, intended to kill and eat him, and would have done so if it hadn't been for the small dog's now deceased best friend, who quickly defended him. Afterwards, the puppy's hero fed him a piece of wild boar, which he recently had killed. That night, after the two dogs ate together, the big dog snuggled up close, protecting and keeping his new puppy friend warm. This is how the small dog that looked like a freak of nature was able to eat and survive over the next several weeks. Then a cold winter storm came that lasted several days, and the big dog could not find any more boars. Both dogs walked together, searching by themselves for several long cold days, without any food. They lost a lot of weight and strength. On one cold, stormy night, after being without shelter for several days, the two dogs finally found a cave. They walked in shivering, snuggling close together as always, after yet another discouraging day without food. The two dogs, both now malnourished, wondered if they would survive the cold night and wake up alive together in the morning.

The big dog soon fell asleep, his stomach rumbling for food. The dog started to close his eyes and fall asleep, when suddenly, his eyes opened up wide, for he thought he saw something jump in and out of the cave. Gently and quietly, he slipped through his big buddy's arms, so as not to wake him. Like a cat, he cautiously crept over to the entrance of the cave to investigate. He stepped outside, looking all around, only to be discouraged, for there was no sign of life. Half starved, the small dog turned around, about to head back into his big buddy's arms, when suddenly a strange lingering scent in the air got his attention. Quickly, he turned his head back around, lifting it up in the air, moving it from side to side, and sniffing. He took three steps to his right, put his nose to the ground, and there smelled fresh urine. His eyes opened wide with the hope of survival. He looked around intently and soon saw some small tracks partially covered by the snow. He followed the tracks over a few small hills, soon finding a large family of rabbits all cuddled up together. Quietly, he crept up to the rabbits, focusing on the biggest one. When he got five feet away, one of the rabbits saw him out of the corner of his eye. The rabbit immediately leaped in the air and ran away. This caused all of the other rabbits to do likewise. The small dog with the short snout chased the big rabbit for hundreds of yards without closing the gap. He was beginning to get very tired, and was running out of steam. Suddenly, he remembered all the times that his big buddy had caught food, keeping him alive. But now his big buddy was unable to do that and could not survive much longer unless he soon had something to eat. The small dog's love for his big buddy gave him the extra little speed needed to catch the rabbit. After resting a few seconds with the dead rabbit in his mouth, the small dog returned to the cave. His big buddy awoke quickly, sitting up, wiggling his tail back and forth as his little friend carried the rabbit over, dropping it off right in front of his face. The big dog licked his little buddy's wrinkled face, expressing gratitude for saving his life. The small dog licked back as if to say, "'Tis my pleasure to save *your* life for a change."

While the big dog ate, the small dog left the cave. He found yet another big rabbit which he chased for several hundred yards. The dog was running out of energy fast, and focused what little he had left into one last attempt. With precise timing, he leaped in the air towards the rabbit, bit the hare's back left leg and held on, literally for his life. Once the rabbit's leg broke, the dog quickly killed this rabbit, just as he had the last. This time, though, he was too tired and hungry to walk, so he caught his breath for a minute, then ate a quarter of the rabbit, which was enough to replenish some of his lost strength. Then he brought the rest of the rabbit back to share with his big buddy, who at the time was looking outside the cave, deeply concerned for him. The dogs shared the rest of the rabbit, and afterwards snuggled up again, but this time their tails wagged, for they were happy this night, having shelter and full stomachs. This is how the two dogs continued to survive over the next three years, by working together as a team. When boar was no more, the small dog with the short snout and wrinkled face, with speed like a fast cat, would provide rodents for the two of them. When rabbits were hard to find, the big dog would catch boar.

After reminiscing about the past, the dog with the short snout became consumed with rage, with lips curled back, and fangs sticking out of his mouth. He slowly turned, looking at the bull that was about to charge out of the alley. The dog with the short snout knew that the bull would be free if he made it to an open space, while he, along with the rest of the dog pack, would probably starve to death because there had been no food to be found in the forest for the past three weeks.

At that moment, the small dog's hunger and rage took over. As the bull started to charge out of the alley, the small dog ran as fast as he possibly could, with every fiber of his being, straight at the bull's face. Jumping in the air, the dog bit the bull right on the most vulnerable part of the bull's body, his nose. With locked jaws, the small dog with the short snout held on like there was no tomorrow as the bull furiously shook his head back and forth, trying desperately to shake this insane freak of nature off of him. But unlike the other dogs, this little freak couldn't be easily shaken off by the bull. A few seconds later, the four big dogs jumped to help their little friend.

Seeing this, the Earl jumped to his feet, his eyes bulging and his jaw dropped, and he stared in disbelief as if he had just seen a ghost. After several minutes of fighting, the bull finally shook off the small dog with the short snout, but only because half of the bull's nose came off along with the dog. The small dog with the short snout flew about twelve feet in the air, doing a flip before perfectly landing on all fours. The bull was just about to spear another dog with one of his horns, when the small dog intervened, springing up and locking his jaws on the remaining half of the bull's nose. Several minutes later, the bull collapsed on the ground, breathing his last breath. The dogs ripped the bull apart, devouring it like the half-starved animals that they were.

The Earl knew that this was his best chance of catching one of these legendary "Hounds of Hell." While the dogs were tearing at the bull, he grabbed his trap and ran toward them. The Earl climbed atop a wall, and looked down over the dogs. Because his favorite dog by far was the small one with the short snout and wrinkled face, the Earl threw his trap over the area where that dog was, but the small dog saw the trap at the last fraction of a second and jumped clear of the net. The Earl, however, managed to trap one of the other dogs in the net, a huge and powerful, female of the Mastiff type, which had evolved from the strongest of dogs that Lord Albert had dropped off. Seeing the huge female in the trap scared the other three big dogs. Before running away, they tore off one last piece of the bull's flesh. The dog with the short snout and wrinkled face stayed behind, trying to help the huge female get free from the net. The Earl calmly came down from the wall. The small dog made eye contact with the Earl, and backed up slowly, growling.

The Earl, maintaining eye contact, slowly walked over to the bull, cut a piece of meat off and held it up for the dog to see and smell while calmly saying, "Come now, this is for thee. Dread not. Ye shall not be harmed." The dog, very hungry, cautiously walked towards the Earl. He was just inches away when he got a good look into the Earl's eyes, and saw through the gateway to his soul that the Earl was a selfish, mean hearted person, with no regard for anyone but himself. The dog also saw the Earl's other hand, the one that wasn't holding the piece of meat. He could tell by the fact that it was wide open and shaking slightly, that the Earl would try to grab him if he were to go for the meat. The small dog turned around, acting as if he were going to run away. Seeing this, the Earl desperately dropped his hands, saying loudly, "NO! Halt! Do not go!" The dog suddenly spun around, unexpectedly jumping at the Earl, ripping the piece of meat right out of his hand before turning around running away. The Earl gave chase, screaming at the top of his lungs, "COME BACK, I charge thee!" But the Earl was just wasting his breath as the small dog with the short snout and wrinkled face quickly ran away, deep into the woods.

It was there he soon ran into another man named Byron Gentry. Byron had very little hair and some permanent burn marks on his face and body, which he had received one night while sleeping at an inn in the town of Rudfield. A drunken man in the next room had staggered, spilling his wine over the wood floor, and then had carelessly knocked over a candle holder with four lit candles which quickly ignited the wine soaked floor. The fire soon engulfed the inn in flames. Byron and his wife Marsha awoke with flames on their bodies. They managed to make it out of the inn together, but unfortunately Marsha, soon died from the massive burns she had received. After Marsha's death, Byron went into a great state of depression. People did not make matters any better by cringing and whispering as they stared at his hideous burns wherever he went. Byron decided to leave civilization. He moved far away from everyone, and had nothing to do with anyone, except for his two sons and grandchildren who would occasionally stop by to visit.

From a short distance away, the small dog with the short snout and wrinkled face watched Byron eat chicken. Byron soon saw the dog licking his lips. For the first time in years, Byron gave a half smile.

"And aren't ye a pleasant sight? I presume thou wouldst like to eat some of this chicken," Byron said as he tore off a piece and held it towards the dog. His right hand remained by his side, in a non-threatening manner. The dog slowly approached Byron, looking deep into his eyes. Unlike what he had seen in the eyes of the Earl, this time the dog saw a kind hearted, loving but injured soul who, like himself, needed a friend. The dog felt comfortable with Byron. Slowly, he walked up and ate the piece of chicken from Byron's hand, allowing Byron to pet him. "Thou hast a very kind spirit and noble eyes; so Noble is the name that I shall give thee." Afterwards, Noble sat next to Byron by the fire, listening to Byron's life story, as Byron had his arm around him shedding tears, baring his soul. Noble licked the tears as he looked at Byron sadly, with his head slightly turned to the right. He was grieved, not only for the loss of his friend earlier, but now for Byron, for he saw the pain in the eyes of this sad and gentle soul.

That night, Noble slept with his back pressed into Byron's chest. Byron's arm was wrapped around him, in much the same way that Noble used to sleep with his big buddy, now deceased. All through the night, a mighty windstorm blew, and continued in the morning. The strong wind knocked down Byron's fence where his lambs lived. The sound of the falling fence woke Noble up. He barked, waking up Byron, who opened his eyes to the site of his frightened lambs running away. Byron quickly jumped to his feet and ran after his flock yelling, "Come back! Come back!" Byron was nowhere near fast enough to stop his lambs from running away. Noble knew what Byron was trying to do. Quickly, he ran past him like the wind, catching up to the flock of lambs, and herding them all back safely to their home. Byron's new helper made sure no more livestock of any kind was lost for the rest of his life.

From Noble, Byron bred several dogs that were just as strange looking and as lighting fast. These dogs that looked like freaks of nature went on to produce the same kind of excellent herding and working dogs that have remained in the Gentry family, even to this day.

On the night of October 30, 1211, William Warne was devastated that Noble, the dog who had the biggest impact on the bull's death, had escaped through his hands. The Earl knew Noble was very special and wanted to breed Noble and reproduce more just like him. He also wanted to try to breed him with a huge and powerful dog, like the female he had dangling in his net, his second most favorite dog of those he had seen that night. The Earl had a theory that breeding could produce the ultimate killing dog, with speed, strength, agility and an awesome bite. The Earl wondered what freak of nature of a dog might come out of that breeding and how such a dog would do fighting against a bull. The Earl was content, though, seeing his second choice dog trapped in his net.

On the other hand, the town of Stamford was not content. They had huge collective chills running down their spines as they watched this monstrosity "Hell Hound" captured and dangling in the Earl's net. They demanded the release of the "Hell Hound" at once, for fear that the "Dogs of Doom" would return, this time devouring the town.

The Earl smiled and waved at the town, replying, "Good people of Stamford, ye are right. May heaven forbid that I should be the cause of the "Dogs of Doom" devouring the wonderful town of Stamford. I shall set this dog free at once. Pray let me take my knife from my bag, so I can cut the "Hell Hound" free from the net." The Earl walked around the corner to where his horse and carriage were, and quickly rode to the captured dog. But instead of setting the dog free, the Earl pulled the huge female into his carriage with all his strength, then whipped his horses and rode away.

The town Priest chased the Earl on foot, yelling after him: "Repent I say, release that hound from hell, lest a curse be bestowed upon you and your seed henceforth!" The Earl continued to ride away, laughing at the Priest. Immediately after the Earl left, the priest and his congregation prayed for protection of their town from the "Hounds of Hell".

Because the Earl was so impressed and entertained by what he had witnessed on October 30, 1211, he tried to recreate exactly what he had seen that night. In doing so, the famous Earl created the legendary sport called bull bating. Every year on the first full moon in October, in his town of Lexington, the Earl would release a large bull, and allow ten half-starved dogs, five large and five small, to chase the bull in an attempt to kill it. Sometimes the bull would win and make it out into the forest, and sometimes the dogs would win, killing the bull. If the dogs were victorious, afterwards the meat of the bull, tenderized by the dogs, would go up for auction to the highest bidder. The whole town, as well as outsiders, would watch and bet a lot of money on this sport. Bull baiting quickly grew and the sport spread to other towns.

Another form of bull baiting was chaining a bull by the neck to a stake in a large tent, then releasing five dogs to attack and try to kill the bull. Whoever was the last standing would be the winner. Bull baiting was one of the most popular sports in medieval times. It was also the bloodiest sport in history.

The bloodlines of the dogs of William Warne and Byron Gentry remained in their families for many generations. The Earl's number one dog was the female that he had caught in Stamford. Through breeding, The Earl produced several other dogs just like that one. But he remained disappointed that he could never find a small dog half as good as Noble.

The famous Earl became a legend, all because he had been so intrigued with the wild stories he had heard about the "Hounds of Hell" of Stamford. His descendants were also very popular. They continued breeding huge fighting dogs with great tenacity. A Warne dog would very seldom, if ever, face defeat against a foe in a fight. The Gentries, unlike the Warnes, remained very low key and humble.

# CHAPTER III
# SPEED AND AGILITY +
# MONSTROSITY STRENGTH

In the year 1540, there lived a direct descendant of the legendary Earl, named Lord Riley Braun Warne. Lord Riley owned some of the world's largest and most powerful dogs. Every day, each dog consumed over ten pounds of raw cow and chicken organs. Seventy percent of this would be expelled as waste, producing an enormous amount of excrement. The average weight of Lord Riley's dogs was about two hundred pounds, which was about twice his own weight. Lord Riley was also short, with long light brown hair and a thick five o'clock shadow. He was a very cruel man with cruel intentions. He trained and bred his dogs to be fighting dogs, just as his relatives had done for several generations before him.

Lord Riley owned some of the best fighting dogs in all of England, which made him a lot of money in dogfights. One day, Lord Riley approached the thirteen and fourteen year olds of the town, asking them to pick up his dogs' leavings, telling them that he would gladly pay them a lot of money. At first, the young people were reluctant. This was a very dirty, smelly job, not to mention that a lot of dog leavings needed to be picked up.

Lord Riley seeing the reluctance said, "Pray let me show ye a little of my pocket change so ye poppets can see what ye could have if ye chose." Lord Riley reached in his pocket, pulled out five gold sovereigns, and tossed them up in the air, while all the youngsters gawked. Seeing this amount of money, the youngsters agreed to pick up after Lord Riley's dogs.

The youngsters spent nearly a full day picking up pounds and pounds of excrement left by Lord Riley's dogs. When the youngsters had completed the task, Lord Riley looked at his yard smiling.

"Job well done. Here is your money. Now go!" But he only handed a measly three pence to one of the lads, who was named Charles Bailey.

Charles replied with a surprised and sad expression, "Forgive me, milord, but did you not say that you would pay us a lot of money?"

Lord Riley answered, "Y-e-s," with a beady-eyed smirk. Charles, with his hand still extended, went on to say, "I do not wish to be disrespectful, milord, but it will be hard to divide these three pence amongst the five of us!" It made Lord Riley chuckle to see the disappointed faces of the youngsters.

"Ungrateful little poppets. This is a lot of money to ye." The youngsters stood there surprised, with sad expressions on their faces, thinking at first that Lord Riley was joking, and was about to hand them the amount of money that they deserved. Lord Riley, annoyed by the youngsters standing around with hurt looks in their eyes, called for his biggest dog. "Oh, George, show these poppets thine appreciation for having picked up all your shite." George came barking and charging at the youngsters, who turned and ran, barely escaping by squeezing through a small hole underneath Lord Riley's fence. Seeing this, Lord Riley laughed even more. The youngsters, on the other hand, were infuriated with Lord Riley and vowed to get even with him someday.

A few days later, a lad named Todd Everson came up with a plan. When they had been at Lord Riley's place, picking up after the dogs, Todd had noticed that Lord Riley's favorite female dog Emerald was in heat, and was kept in a kennel all by herself. But Todd knew a lad named Thomas Gentry with a lively little mutt named Rascal. Todd's plan was to borrow Rascal and mate him with Emerald. Rascal looked like a freak of nature, having a pushed in nose and bottom lip that extended out over the top lip. Just about everyone who saw Rascal agreed that he was the weirdest looking creature that they had ever seen. For that reason, Rascal was looked down upon and treated like an outcast, as was his master, Thomas. Thomas was very shy and different from the rest of the youngsters. Whenever he and Rascal passed by the youngsters of the town, they ridiculed both dog and master.

Usually, Todd start the teasing by pointing and saying things like, "Look! Tis the two bloody freaks of nature!" This was followed by the rest of the youngsters laughing and making other hurtful comments. Hanging his head in shame, Thomas would run away, accompanied by his dog. However, the person who hurt Thomas the most was a girl named Emily Sinclair. Emily was a stunning beauty, with long blonde hair and feminine curves. She didn't make any comments about Rascal, but would laugh like the others, along with her boy friend Todd and the rest of the youngsters. Todd could see in Thomas' eyes that he had a crush on his girlfriend. Todd was very insecure about his nose, which was huge, and his hair, which was straight, ash blond, and messy. Thomas, on the other hand, had nice dark brown curly hair, with an appealing turned-up nose. Because Todd knew that Thomas was a much nicer person and much better looking than he was himself, he deliberately belittled Rascal and Thomas in front of Emily. Thomas thought that Emily was the most beautiful girl he had ever seen, especially now at fourteen with his hormones kicking in at full force. When Todd influenced Emily to laugh at Thomas and Rascal, it hurt Thomas more than the ridicule of everyone else combined.

However, Todd was not Thomas' biggest enemy. That title was reserved for Lord Riley's nephew, Vivian. Like his father Sherman III, Vivian was short and slender, with dark brown hair and eyes. Vivian was unaware that his father was a contract killer. If someone was discreet and able to pay a fortune, Sherman III was the best money could buy. Vivian was a demented young lad, mainly due to his heartless father. The first time Vivian saw Rascal, he pointed him out to his bullying acquaintances.

"Look ye there, mates, at the bloody freak of nature" Vivian said laughing hysterically. "'Tis the ugliest looking creature ever I have seen!" Hearing this, Thomas, kept quiet and tried to avoid a confrontation by walking away from Vivian, but he quickly followed, along with his acquaintances, taunting, "You, lad, your dog is so ugly that he makes the ugliest of bitches look good, including your mother!" Thomas took deep breaths, walking faster as he ignored Vivian's comments and laughter. "You! 'Tis you I am addressing, you lover of freaks! Do not walk away." (Naturally Thomas kept walking.) "I shall not be ignored!" Immediately after Vivian said this, he pointed Rascal out to Angus, his fighting dog, commanding, "Kill!" Frightened at hearing this, Thomas turned around and saw a gigantic, mean, fighting dog running at Rascal in attack mode.

"Run, Rascal!" Thomas yelled quickly. He did not have to repeat himself. Rascal, just as frightened, turned and ran as fast as he could, while Angus chased him. Vivian laughed at how scared Rascal was.

"Why did you command your dog to leave and thereby spoil my dog's fun?" Vivian said with a devilish smirk. "He wanted only to get better acquainted with your dog and fight with him in play." Thomas, very angry, looked at Vivian.

"I heard you tell your dog to attack mine!" Vivian tried to act innocent, holding his hands with his palms open facing up.

"I did not say that." He chuckled as he replied.

"I heard you." Thomas harshly responded.

"Do you call me a liar?" Vivian asked as he walked toward Thomas with his friends.

"Pray let my dog, and me, alone. We have done nothing to you," Thomas pleaded as he walked backwards.

"But you have done." Vivian told him as he walked up to Thomas' face. "You and the ugly aspect of your dog disturb the eye!" Vivian signaled his big bully acquaintances Derrick and James to seize Thomas, which they quickly did. They twisted Thomas' arms behind him, as Vivian slapped Thomas across the face.

"Ouch! Have mercy, pray." Thomas moaned, not so much from the pain of the slap, but from the feeling that his arms were about to break off from being twisted behind him. Vivian smiled as Thomas moaned with pain.

"Right now methinks you would change your dog for mine." Vivian arrogantly stated, "and would thus escape this present predicament. However, you cannot. Your ugly, useless mongrel will never be able to defeat Angus! Nor will any of his seed." Vivian paused to slap Thomas a few more times. "Ye two are pathetic and weak, and will never amount to anything, unlike Angus who is strong!" Angus had just returned, and as Vivian said this, he petted Angus on the head. "His seed will produce many more powerful fighting dogs, which will enable me someday to buy and rule the land, making me rich, just like my uncle, Lord Riley!" After saying this, Vivian punched Thomas in the stomach with all his might. Thomas had the wind momentarily knocked out of him, while Vivian sprained his wrist, an injury Vivian tried to pass off as if he was fine. But everyone could tell by how he immediately grabbed his wrist for a second that he was hurt.

"Ye two can now let him go." Vivian told Derrick and James with a hint of pain in his voice. After twisting Thomas' arm one last time, Vivian's friends let Thomas go. As they turned and walked away, Vivian chuckled as he spoke to Angus. "'Tis glad ye are back. Did that ugly dog make a nice little meal?" Thomas was still on the ground, moaning from the pain in his arms. Rascal soon came to his side and stood over him licking his face.

Thomas smiled, knowing his dog was safe. He pet Rascal, saying, "I care not what anybody says! I would have no other dog but thee." Thomas had no friends except for his dog Rascal. He only had one acquaintance, Charles Bailey. Charles had dirty blonde hair, and like Thomas, he was very handsome. Charles' parents were good friends with Thomas' family. His father, Edgerrin, was the best friend of Thomas' uncle Robert. Robert's wife had died of gangrene five years earlier. Edgerrin proved his friendship to Robert by standing by him in Robert's time of need. The Gentry's and the Bailey's have been attending the same church for several years. Charles would sometimes see Thomas on Sunday mornings and greet him, which would normally be the extent of their conversation. However, when Charles was around his other friends, and Thomas and Rascal were in sight, Thomas and Rascal would be ridiculed, but instead of sticking up for them, Charles kept quiet and kind of chuckled along with his friends.

Over the next few days, Todd kept an eye on Lord Riley's manor, waiting for him to leave, which he finally did, to attend an underground bloody dogfight. Lord Riley took a couple of his fighting dogs and left for the next few hours. Luckily for the youngsters of the town, it was Sunday morning and the Gentry's were at church. So Todd and his friends opened the Gentry's gate, letting Rascal out. Rascal raised his head up in the air, and moved it right to left, soon locking onto the scent of Emerald. Rascal could smell Emerald a mile away and went running towards Lord Riley's manor, followed by the youngsters of the town. When Rascal and the youngsters of the town arrived at Lord Riley's manor, Emerald was in her cage. At first, when Emerald saw the youngsters, she barked and growled at them, until they gave Emerald some raw liver. She then accepted them. The young people quickly opened Emerald's cage door and let her out. Rascal and Emerald were in lust at first scent. Unfortunately, because of the huge size difference between them, it was hard for Rascal and Emerald to mate on their own. So, the youngsters of the town picked up Rascal and threw him on top of Emerald, towards her rear end. Rascal was able to wrap his front paws around Emerald's lower back, mating with her for about half and hour, successfully impregnating her. All the young people watching this rolled around on the ground, crying with laughter at this funny sight. Knowing how angry Lord Riley would be when he found out that his best female dog was impregnated by a strange looking mutt, a lad named Lawrence was looking around nervously, and saw Lord Riley approaching from a distance with his dogs. Lawrence quickly stopped laughing. He got up, and threw a little piece of liver back in Emerald's cage, luring her back in to it. The kids quickly closed the cage. They took Rascal and quickly squeezed underneath the fence just before Lord Riley could see them in his yard. The faces of the youngsters were red and their cheeks were puffed out from the effort to control their laughter. They walked past Lord Riley, acting as if Rascal was their dog, and they were taking him for a walk. Lord Riley, seeing the kids, smiled at them sarcastically saying, "Hallo, have you returned to pick up more of my dog's shite? Ha, ha, ha!" Lord Riley looked at Rascal, with a cringing face. "Oh, by the way, your dog is the ugliest I have ever seen in all of my days. I would not be caught dead with an ugly, useless dog such as that, unlike my dogs, the most powerful, best fighting dogs in the world," Lord Riley said while patting George on top of his head. Then Lord Riley thought, *"Wait a minute, I do think I have seen this ugly dog somewhere before, but where?"* Lord Riley put his hand to his chin with his head lowered, thinking, *"Nay, perhaps not!"* The young people of the town didn't say a word, but just smiled and chuckled a little with their hands covering their mouths to keep them from laughing hysterically as they continued to walk by. When the youngsters were far away from Lord Riley, they laughed hysterically, rolling around on the ground again, not paying any attention to Rascal, who ran away. Afterwards, the youngsters searched for Rascal for a while.

"I warrant he is probably already home," Todd said, not giving a damn. "We do waste our time away out here." The youngsters soon gave up. Halfway home, Rascal heard his master, who was out looking and calling for him. Rascal instantly ran and jumped in Thomas' arms,

"Thou art alright, thank the good Lord! I do not know what I would do if anything should befall me best mate," Thomas told Rascal as he hugged him.

# CHAPTER IV
# BIRTH OF A LEGEND

A few weeks later, Lord Riley was the happiest man in all of England because Emerald, his favorite female dog, was pregnant. Of course, Lord Riley thought the sire was his favorite male dog, George. One month later, when Emerald gave birth to five puppies, Lord Riley was very pleased at first, but was a little surprised that the puppies weren't a lot bigger. "Oh well," Lord Riley said to himself. "With Emerald and George as their parents, these dogs will soon grow into giants too." However, they did not. About two weeks later, Lord Riley was convinced that George was not the father of these puppies. He said to himself, "How in the world could this be?" Then suddenly, while looking at one of the male puppies, Lord Riley remembered the youngsters of the town who had picked the leavings of his dogs. He remembered them chuckling while they were walking a dog near his manor. He could see the resemblance between the boy's dog and Emerald's puppies. Lord Riley slapped his face with both hands, realizing that this was a trick to pay him back because he hadn't paid the youngsters what they deserved for picking up after his dog's. Furious, Lord Riley ran down the street, screaming for vengeance. He found the young lads of the town playing together. Then at the top of his voice, he yelled, "I will kill ye, ye bloody sons of bitches!" Lord Riley had no problem in taking advantage of other people, but if anyone tried to take advantage of him, he would go crazy. Lord Riley threw rocks at the youngsters, but luckily for them, had a bad aim and missed. A couple of constables happened to be nearby at the time and saw Lord Riley throwing rocks. The constables instantly tackled Lord Riley, arresting him before any of the youngsters were injured. The constables then brought Lord Riley before the judge.

"Oh, 'tis you again!" the judge said in disgust, looking at Lord Riley and shaking his head. "Lord Riley, have you still not paid your taxes?"

One of the Constables explained to the judge, "Your honor, Lord Riley is not here for late taxes this time. He hath been brought before you for forcefully throwing rocks at youngsters." The judge, eyes narrowed, raised his gavel over his head and slammed it hard against the bench.

"ERRR! I hereby sentence Lord Riley Braun Warne to spend six weeks in jail, for his indecent acts and boorish conduct!" After the judge sentenced Lord Riley, he stood up and mumbled to himself with disgust, as he walked away "Were Riley not a lord, I would have him hanged!"

Lord Riley was taken to jail by the constables immediately after he was sentenced. He promised the prison guards at jail free admittance to his bull baiting events. The prison guards treated Lord Riley like royalty. Therefore his stay was an easy one. He was given three full fancy meals a day, all the sleep he desired and never had to lift a finger to do any chores. Unlike the other prisoners, who had to work long strenuous hours, with limited sleep and without three full meals a day.

When released, Lord Riley ran home, terrified his dogs might all be dead from starvation. But because Lord Riley had left his manor in pure rage, he hadn't paid attention to closing his gate properly, so his dogs were able to get out and hunt for themselves. When Lord Riley finally got home, he saw piles of dog leavings and wild boar scraps all over his yard. He checked on all his dogs and was greatly relieved that they were all right. Lord Riley then turned towards the pups, with anger in his eyes.

"Thy father is a disgrace to the canine species! Ye shall all die!" Emerald, knowing Lord Riley's intentions, growled at him. Lord Riley knew that he could not kill the puppies there in front of Emerald without her someday turning on him. Therefore, he grabbed a couple of pieces of raw pig and lured the puppies deep into the woods, near Hellhound Forest, where for the past three hundred years only the strongest dogs had survived. Having reached the deep woods, Lord Riley took out his sword and raised it over his head. He was just about to kill all of the puppies, but then, for the first time in several years, his heart melted a little. He looked at the puppies and noticed how cute they all looked playing together. Even Lord Riley, with all the evil in his heart, could not kill them. He turned and started to walk away. At the last second, Lord Riley turned back around again and walked over to the puppies. He took one of the two strongest males, the one that he thought might soon be a decent dog to use for training one of his fighting dogs. When Lord Riley took the puppy, the others were all very sad to see their litter mate leave. The big puppy in Lord Riley's arms looked sadly back at his brothers and sister as he was being carried away. He loved his littermates and knew that they needed him to help hunt if they were to survive. The pups were also very sad that their brother was being taken away, especially the big puppy that was left. He was going to miss his brother the most. The two big pups really had fun wrestling hard with each other. They couldn't wrestle as hard with their other littermates because the other pups would get hurt. The big puppy that was left followed his brother as he was being carried away, crying behind him. Lord Riley heard the pup whine, and turned around to look, annoyed.

"Get back to your littermates! Die with them, you bloody little son of a bitch!" said Lord Riley, as he started to kick the puppy. As he swung his leg, the puppy that Lord Riley was carrying bit him on the shoulder, in defense of his brother. "Ouch!" Lord Riley screamed, as his foot missed the puppy by just an inch. The pup in Lord Riley's arms held his bite as his brother ran away uninjured. Lord Riley had to pry the pup's little jaws off of him. The pup tried to attack again, but Lord Riley raised him far above his head. As the pup squirmed, Lord Riley yelled in pain and said, "Time to die!" Just before Lord Riley was going to splatter the puppy against the ground, he looked at the blood on his shoulder and the teeth marks and stopped himself. "Hmm, very impressive for a bloody little pup, especially for thy age and size. Look thee, out of my rage I did very nearly kill thee just now, in which event thou wouldst have been better off." Chuckling, Lord Riley flicked the blood off his shoulder into the pup's face. "This blood and mark that thou hast inflicted upon me shall not compare to the amount of suffering and bleeding that shall be inflicted upon thee. For when thou art a little older, thou shalt be put in the pit against my best fighting dog, in which circumstance thou shalt surely suffer a dreadful death, but that will, I hope, help my fighting dog to become an even better fighter!" Lord Riley continued walking, carrying the pup by the scruff of the neck, because the pup was trying to bite him. He named the dog Tiny because he had never before had an eight-week-old pup that was this small.

Lord Riley left the other puppies, three male and one female, to fend for themselves in the forest. After a while, the puppies became very hungry. Nearby, a huge wild dog was eating a deer that he recently had killed. The puppies watched from a distance, licking their lips. They tried to hide in some shrubs near a large hole, but the wild dog noticed the puppies. When he was finished eating, he bit off a big piece of venison from the deer, and carried it over to the half-starved puppies. When the pups saw this gigantic wild dog walk their way, they ran and hid in the hole. The wild dog dropped the piece of venison near the pups, turned and ran away. As soon as the wild dog left, the pups came out and devoured the venison.

The next day, the same gigantic dog and his wild dog mates noticed a bear catching fish from the river. The wild dogs waited until the bear had his back completely turned away from his pile of fish, then the huge wild dog crept up, grabbing the largest fish and ran. Furious, the bear chased after him. While this was happening, the other wild dogs took the rest of the bear's fish. After the bear gave up chasing the gigantic dog, he returned to his favorite fishing spot only to find all of his fish gone. Out of rage, the bear stood up, looking up at the sky and growling as loudly as he could. He tried to catch more fish, but it was not the right time of day for fishing. The sun had just gone down, so the bear did not have any more luck. The bear raised his head, stood up hungry and growled out of rage because his dinner had been stolen.

The huge wild dog carried his fish close to where the puppies were. He tore a big piece of fish off for the puppies. The gigantic dog sat down and started eating. The female puppy, which was the bravest, cautiously came out of the hole, sat down next to the gigantic dog, and ate next to him. When the other puppies saw this, they also cautiously came out and ate next to the gigantic dog. When they were all finished eating, the gigantic dog stood up and started to leave. The female puppy gave a little bark. The gigantic dog turned around. The female puppy ran up to the gigantic dog and licked him on the nose as if to say thanks, then turned and walked back to her brothers. The gigantic dog said through a soft growl to her.

"Fret not. I know that you are frightened out here, but I will protect and keep you from harm." Then the huge dog ran to join his pack, which was howling at the moon.

The next morning, the puppies were awakened by the sound of gunshots. There were hunters in the area. They were shooting at anything that moved. The pack of dogs would leave that area, never to return. The gigantic wild dog knew that the puppies could not survive alone, on their own. So, just before leaving, he went to where the puppies were hiding and with his mouth, gently picked up the female puppy by the neck. He looked sadly at the rest of the puppies as if to say, "Sorry, my friends, to leave you here, but I can not take any more of you with me." The gigantic dog turned and ran like the wind, trying to rejoin his pack. Unfortunately, the gigantic dog heard a lot of gunshots in the direction of his pack's location. He knew then that he would never see his pack again. The only chance that he and the pup had to survive was to run in a completely different direction, so he did so, for several miles without stopping. Finally, when the gigantic dog and pup were safe and far away from the hunters, he gently put her down. The average puppy would have been badly injured by being carried for so long and held so firmly. However, because of the unusual amount of wrinkled skin that this puppy had, she was unharmed. She was very lucky, for this gigantic dog loved her very much and would die for her.

Meanwhile, however, her three brothers didn't have anybody watching over them. They were three pups on their own. The hunter's dogs soon came by, and the pups hid in their hole the moment they saw them. The hunter's dogs smelled the pups there and barked. The hunters came and looked inside the hole, but didn't see anything.

Therefore, they said, "Oh, 'tis no doubt a small rodent in there. Let us leave and go find some bigger prey to kill, and perhaps we will return afterwards."

The hunters took their dogs and left, but the pups stayed in their hole for a few more hours because they were afraid. When they started to get hungry, they came out looking for food. It didn't take long before the big pup smelled fresh rat urine. He gave a little bark, notifying his two brothers. They knew that the rat was close by. Quietly, they walked through the woods until they found the rat sitting near a tree. The three inexperienced pups ignorantly charged at the rat. The rat saw and heard the pups and took off running. The pups spent the next four hours searching for the rat before finally finding him again, just before the sun went down, in the middle of a field. The pups knew that this rat was much faster than they were. Their only chance of catching him was to work together as a team. So the pups split up around the rat. The first pup charged at the rat, causing him to run close to the second pup. The second pup chased the rat toward the big pup, which was hiding in some bushes near a large hole. The big pup came out just as the rat approached. The rat tried to jump over him and run into the hole, but the big pup sprang up in the air at the same time, biting the rat on the end of his tail. The two came crashing to the ground. The rat kicked the pup in the face but the pup held on. The rat tried to bite the big pup. As the rat's teeth scraped the pup's face, the second pup bit the rat on the neck, protecting his big brother. A second later, he was joined by the first pup, who attacked the rat's stomach. The three pups soon killed the rat. They went to sleep that night on a full stomach.

For the next six days, the pups continued to hunt rodents. Sometimes the pups would catch them, and sometimes the rodents would get away. Over the next six days, the pups never went to sleep hungry. On the seventh day, the pups killed a giant rat. Immediately afterwards, a small wild boar smelled the kill that happened to be in the area. He wanted to eat the rat himself, the wild boar charged at the puppies just as they were about to eat. The puppies saw the boar charging at them out of the corner of their eyes, and tried to run away. But the pups were not as fast as the wild boar. The boar opened his mouth and was just about to bite one of the pups, but the big pup bit the boar on the left side of the throat, and held on. A second later, the pup that had almost got bitten locked his jaws on the boar's nose and held on. In the next second, the third pup bit the boar on the right side of the throat and held on. All three pups kept holding on and were swung all around by the boar. The pup on the boar's right side was bashed against a tree, but still somehow managed to hang on, while the pup that was biting the boar's nose was smashed against the ground and scraped by the tusks but somehow he also managed to hang on. After several minutes of fighting, the wild boar collapsed on the ground, close to death. The big pup left the fight a very lucky dog. He was badly bruised with some slight cuts, but no broken bones. Unfortunately his two brothers weren't so fortunate. They each had several broken bones and had extremely bad bruises. They were too badly injured to walk. The big pup licked his two brothers' wounds. He ripped off a piece of boar's meat and tried to put it in his brothers' mouths to feed them. But his brothers were so badly injured that they did not wish to eat, and soon like the boar, both died. The big pup cried himself to sleep that night alone over the loss of his two brothers.

# CHAPTER V
# ONLY THE STRONG SURVIVE

Two days later, Thomas woke up to find that his dog Rascal had died of natural causes in his sleep. Rascal had lived to be one hundred and nine years old, in dog years of course. Thomas took Rascal's death very hard. He lay next to his best friend, hugging and crying over him. Thomas' parents, for the first time since Thomas was a baby, were awakened by Thomas' crying. They looked at each other deeply concerned, both thinking that Rascal's time had finally came. They quickly got out of bed and went to their son.

"Oh no, my poor child!" Mrs. Gentry said, seeing her son crying and holding Rascal dead in his arms. Hearing his mother, Thomas turned and looked at her, as tears poured out of his eyes. His mother, seeing Rascal dead and her son distressed, quickly ran over to him. She got down on her knees and cried as she held him.

"We are so sorry, son," Mr. Gentry said as he walked towards Thomas, gently putting his hands on his son's shoulders. "Death of a loved one is never easy. But always remember, my son, there is someone up above who hath a plan and purpose for everything. It may take time, but put thy trust in the Lord, and the Lord will heal thy soul."

Hearing his father's words and feeling his hands on him, Thomas turned and glanced at him, with a face wet with tears.

"Rascal is one lucky dog, son," Mr. Gentry went on to say, as he massaged Thomas' shoulders. "Right now I warrant Rascal is entering the pearly gates, with a wagging tail." Thomas stopped crying for a moment, as he looked up at his father.

"Do you believe that, truly?" Thomas asked, wiping his wet face.

"Most assuredly I do, my son. When next thou shalt see Rascal again, he shall give thee the biggest tongue washing thou hast ever received!" Thomas turned towards Rascal, breaking away from his mother's embrace, wrapping his arms around Rascal, crying again.

"Rascal did live a good long happy life, the kind of life most dogs only dream about," Mrs. Gentry told Thomas, with her hand on his back and tears in her eyes, for she felt her son's pain. "Both thy father and I do love thee greatly, my son. If ever thou hast need of us, we will offer thee what comfort we can." Mrs. and Mr. Gentry knew their son wanted to be alone. So both gently kissed their son on the head and quietly turned, walking away. When Thomas' eyes became very sore from crying, he dried his face and looked towards the heavens praying.

"My thanks, O Lord, for giving me such a wonderful companion. Never have I asked for a miracle until now!" Thomas paused a second, taking in a deep breath, then bent over hugging and crying over Rascal again, as he continued praying. "Dear Lord, please bring Rascal's spirit back."

After this prayer, Thomas put his head next to Rascal's heart, weeping as he listened for several minutes. Rascal's heart, however, did not begin to beat again. "Why hast thou forsaken me?" Thomas asked with a raised voice, as he stood up with his head hung low. Thomas, feeling abandoned, took a long walk to be by himself. After hours of shedding tears and miles of staring off into the horizon while he walked, reminiscing about all the good times he had shared with his best friend, Thomas heard rocks being thrown, and laughter. He went over to the source of the noise to investigate. He hid behind a tree and saw Derrick and James Tate. They were huge brothers whose hearts had been turned to stone by their alcoholic father, who abused them both physically and mentally. The boys were throwing rocks at the dead boar that the three puppies had killed a few days earlier. After throwing several rocks at the boar, Derrick saw the two dead puppies a short distance away.

"Brother, look thee at those pups. They look very like that stupid, ugly dog of Thomas Gentry! Methinks they are dead though, but just to be sure . . . .." James said, throwing a rock at one of the dead puppies. Seeing this, Thomas quickly came out from behind the tree, running towards the puppies and yelling,

"Halt! Pray leave off throwing rocks. It is not certain that these puppies are dead!"

James responded with a devilish smile as he continued to throw more rocks at the pups.

"Yes, you are right, we do not know." Thomas approached the two puppies. Derrick picked up a rock, and cocked his arm back in the direction of Thomas.

"Never tell us what we can and cannot do, you little freak." After saying this, Derrick threw the rock in his hand at Thomas, hitting him on the shoulder. Thomas instantly fell to the ground, bawling like a baby, not really because of the rock, but mainly because of the thought of his dead best friend, and the two little dead puppies next to him, which resembled Rascal. James was also about to throw a rock at Thomas. However, seeing Thomas on the ground bawling like a baby influenced him to drop the rock in his hand and motion toward Thomas, waving his hand to the side and looking disgusted as he shook his head.

"You are one pitiful little freak!" Derrick said, shaking his head, looking at Thomas in pity. "Come James, let this pitiful little freak be with his dead, bloody mates." They both turned, walking away laughing. Meanwhile, Thomas rolled on his back and was lying on the ground, staring up at the sky and crying out.

"Good Lord, me best mate is gone. I do wish so badly that I was with him right now. Please help me, someday, to find another companion half as special as Rascal." Thomas turned his head, looking at the two dead puppies. With tears in his eyes he continued praying. "Also God, please grant these two adorable pups a place in Thy kingdom above, and if there are any more of them out there, I pray Thou wilt protect them." Immediately after saying this prayer, Thomas turned his head to his right and saw Rascal's distinct blue left eye, and brown right eye looking back at him. Rascal's son, who had survived, cautiously approached Thomas. The puppy shared Thomas' pain and, watching through some thick bushes, had seen how Thomas had tried to protect his two brothers from the two cruel lads. Thomas, seeing the puppy, stopped crying and held out his hand saying, "Tis alright mate. Come here. I shall never harm thee." The pup and Thomas both felt an instant bond between them and could tell that each needed the other to help mend his broken heart. With his head down, the pup continued slowly walking towards Thomas. Thomas lay on the ground with tears across his face. When the puppy approached Thomas, he started licking the tears off of Thomas' face. Thomas gave a little smile, seeing and holding in his arms this beautiful puppy with Rascal's eyes, short snout and wrinkles. His tears of sorrow were slowly replaced with tears of joy. Thomas was convinced that this puppy had Rascal's spirit in him. He looked back up in the sky saying, "O Lord, my thanks, for returning me best mate to me so soon!" Thomas picked the puppy up, giving him a kiss right on the lips. Then he immediately pulled the puppy away, spitting with a sour look. "I do love thee, pup. However, thou hast horrible breath. What hast thou eaten?" After asking this, Thomas smelled a rancid scent. He looked near the dead pig and saw half of a rat. He continued to spit all the way home as he carried his new friend. Upon arriving home, Thomas introduced the puppy to his parents. They instantly loved the pup and welcomed him as their new family member. Both Thomas' parents were shocked and commented about how much this new puppy looked like Rascal.

"What dost thou think to name him?" Thomas' mother asked. Thomas looked carefully at the pup.

"I do not know just yet. I am still thinking about it." At that moment, the pup saw a skunk and ran right up to it fearlessly. Thomas seeing this yelled, "NO!" as he grabbed the pup, quickly pulling him away from the skunk. Thomas scared the skunk, which ending up spraying him as he turned around right on the back of his shirt. Thomas' parents both broke out in laughter.

"Son, never have I seen a dog more daring than this new pup." Thomas's mother said as she held her nose.

Thomas took off his shirt saying, "You have just given me an idea! My new pup's name shall be Dare."

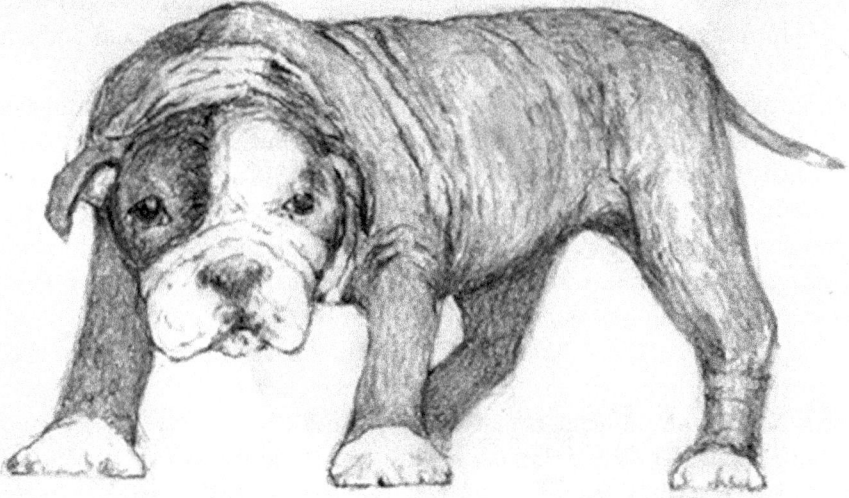

Pup approaching Thomas for the first time.

# CHAPTER VI
# BULLIES VERSES BULLDOG

Seven months went by. The friendship between Thomas and Dare continued to grow, and the two were virtually inseparable. They did everything together. They went fishing together, swam together, played tug of war with a rope together, and did just about everything else. Dare grew up very strong and agile. He lived and breathed for his master, Thomas. Dare would give his life for his master or his master's parents, with no hesitation and without thinking twice, if the situation were to arise.

One day, Dare and Thomas were coming home from a very successful day of fishing, with Thomas carrying the day's catch, when Dare started barking ferociously to the right at some bushes up the hill.

"What is wrong, mate?" asked Thomas, as he looked up the hill, in the direction where Dare was barking. "If anyone is up there, pray come out." Derrick and James Tate soon came out from behind the bushes where Dare was barking at, with a couple of knives in their hands.

"My, my, what do we have here?" Derrick said, as he took in a dramatic, deep breath, smelling the fish. "I do think it looks like we will have some nice fresh fish tonight for dinner! Is that not so, James?"

James nodded his head, licking his lips looking at the fish, answering, "I wager thou art right, brother."

Thomas held the fish close to his chest. "This fish belongs to me and to my family! If it is fish you want, go catch your own!"

"Shut your mouth!" Derrick abruptly interrupted, waving his knife back and forth while looking at Dare, who was barking at him. "I also do advise you to shut Rover up, and give us our fish now! Otherwise, your life as well as Rover's life will be at an end!"

Thomas, with his head hung low, dropped the fish saying, "Come Dare, let us go home. Thy life is worth more than all the fish in the world." At first, Dare walked close by his master's side, but soon turned and watched Derrick and James smile as they walked towards the fish, which Dare and his master had caught. Dare thought, *"There is no way that I am going to let them bully my master and take our supper."* So Dare ran over to the string of fish. Right at the moment when James was bent over in the process of picking up the string of fish, Dare snatched the fish right out of James's hands and took off running. Thomas followed, shouting after him. "Come back Dare! Come back!" But Dare kept on running, as James and Derrick chased after them shouting, "Ye two are dead when we catch ye!" However, the brothers could not catch Thomas and his dog, and soon gave up. James, sweating, collapsed on the ground, taking a minute to catch his breath. He looked up at Derrick with fear in his eyes. "Now we must tell our father that we did not catch any fish."

Derrick replied bent over catching his breath. "Must thou remind me?"

Thomas chased Dare all the way home. Thomas' mother was outside. A huge smile came upon her face when she saw Dare running with the fish he was carrying.

"Good husband, do thou come here and see the fish our son hath caught and the clever trick he hath taught his dog to do!" Thomas' father came outside, clapping his hands while he watched Dare carry the full string of fish in his mouth.

"I am very proud of thee, my son. Thou art an excellent fisherman, and thou hast even taught thy dog to work for thee! I am most impressed, my son!" Mr. Gentry said, patting Thomas on the shoulder.

Meanwhile Derrick and James were just arriving home. When they opened the door, the first thing they saw was their hefty father with his dark beard and long, messy gray hair, holding a bottle of wine and looking irritated.

"Well my sons, and where's the fish that ye promised to catch for supper?" Derrick cringed as he answered.

"Sorry, father, 'twas a bad day for fishing; Nobody caught anything today."

Mr. Tate finished drinking his wine, shaking his head in disgust. "Oh! Is that so!" His voice reflected his fury, "Then how is it that I saw Thomas' dog carry home a full string of fish? Even a stupid dog knows how to fish better than ye two buffoons!" Before James answered his father, he swallowed and started to sweat from fear, knowing that their father would now be even angrier with them, because they had just been caught lying.

"Well, father, 'tis because Thomas and his dog happened to be in a fortunate spot today."

"Stop lying to me!" Mr. Tate responded, as he slapped James across the face. "Ye lazy bastards should have gotten out of bed sooner! That way ye might have caught something! However, 'tis for the laziness of the two of ye that I must go to bed hungry again!"

"We are sorry, father!" James responded with his fingers touching the blood from his lips, "Tomorrow we shall get out of bed earlier. We shall come home with fish tomorrow, I do promise you." Mr. Tate sat down with closed eyes, putting one hand on his head for a second before replying.

"I have heard this story and thy lies for a very long time now. 'Tis obvious that ye took no heed when I told ye how to fish. Therefore, ye both should befriend Thomas and go fishing with him. Learn how he catches fish." Hearing this, both lads clenched their fists with rage.

"We do not need that bloody bastard to teach us how to fish! Besides, we almost caught a giant fish today, but at the last second, he escaped. But by then, we had lost much valuable time."

Their father sighed at James's comments. "Oh I pray thee, leave off! Dost thou think me a fool?" he said, pacing back and forth and waving his hands in the air. "'Tis constantly I do hear these pathetic tales about the one that got away from ye two buffoons. I do not give a damn about stories. 'Tis fish I care about! So bring me some!"

Early the next morning, Thomas left to go fishing, but without Dare. When Dare sadly watched his master leave, his tail was still. Dare always went fishing with his master. However, Thomas wasn't going to take any chances of running into Derrick and James with Dare along, for fear they might hurt him. Thomas did not have much luck that morning. He only caught a couple of fish. His mind wasn't much on fishing. One reason for this was he missed his best friend, who was always by his side. So Thomas quit early that morning, deeply depressed, remembering the sad look that Dare gave him when he had left without him.

While Thomas was fishing, Dare tried to jump the eight-foot fence so he could be with his master. However, he kept coming about one foot short of clearing it, so he gave up, at least until he heard Derrick talking to James as they walked by.

"Brother, I do declare that we shall take the fish from that little freak today, and no person nor dog shall get in our way." After hearing this, Dare tried to jump the fence again, but he was still about a six inches too short. After five attempts, Dare rested to catch his breath. At this moment, Derrick and James approached Thomas as he was on his way home.

"Hey there, little freak. Where is your mate, the bloody freak of nature?" Derrick asked, hitting the knuckles of one hand against the palm of his other hand. Thomas kept quiet and kept walking. James grabbed Thomas, stopping him, putting Thomas in a headlock, as Derrick punched Thomas in the stomach causing him to scream in pain.

"OUGH!" Dare heard his master scream. Knowing his master was in trouble caused Dare to have twice his normal strength. Quickly, he ran towards the fence growling, this time effortlessly jumping over it. Dare then ran like the wind to defend his master, who at that moment was on the ground, trying to catch his breath. Derrick picked up Thomas' pair of fish.

"I shall be taking this now!" Derrick said with a pissed off look. "'Tis such a pity that this is all you caught today!" Thomas remained quiet on the ground. Derrick grabbed Thomas' collar, looking down at him, with his fist pulled back, ready to punch again.

Raising his voice, he said, "I do advise you to get your lazy arse out of bed earlier tomorrow to catch us more fish than this! Otherwise, next time, we shall beat your arse bloody and shall eat your dog, that freak of nature!" Thomas closed his eyes, trembling with rage. Derrick thought Thomas was scared and was about to cry. He slapped Thomas on the back of his head. "Stop shaking like a chicken!" Derrick said, chuckling. "Open up your eyes and look at me, you little cry baby!" Thomas slowly looked up at Derrick with eyes like a roaring lion, ready to devour his prey. Thomas no longer felt any pain because of what Derrick had said. Thomas rose to his feet, taking a deep breath, then with all of his strength, punched Derrick right in the jaw, knocking him to the ground. Thomas was just about to connect his foot with Derrick's face, but at the last second, James stopped Thomas by grabbing him from behind, and putting him in a full nelson. Derrick got up, spitting blood out of his mouth onto Thomas' face. "I do declare you have just made the biggest mistake of your life," Derrick said while taking a couple of steps towards Thomas, who yelled out, concerned with only his dog, not himself.

"If you hurt my dog in any way, you will have to kill me! If you do not, I swear to God almighty I shall make you wish you were never born!"

Derrick shook his head responding, "Ha, strong words for somebody who's about to meet God, if He indeed exists." Derrick pulled his arm back and was just about to hit Thomas, when Dare came out of nowhere, grabbing Derrick's back collar with his teeth and threw him to the ground headfirst. Dare then turned and stared James right in the eyes, growling and showing his massive razor sharp fangs. Seeing this, Thomas looked at his dog in disbelief, with his mouth open. For until now, he had only seen Dare as a nice dog that loved everything and everyone, not this raging beast that looked like it was about to kill.

Seeing Dare in this state, James instantly let go of Thomas and remained still as a board, while softly saying, "Nice doggie, nice dog." However, Derrick wasn't as smart. He reached into his pocket and pulled out his knife, intending to stab Dare with it. Seeing the knife, Thomas screamed, "Dare, look out!" and tried to grab the knife out of Derrick's hand in Dare's defense. Derrick, seeing Thomas charging at him, shifted his attention to Thomas and moved to stab Thomas across the right arm. Just as the blade was about to make contact with Thomas' arm, Dare bit Derrick's hand, causing him to scream in pain and drop his knife. Dare then sprung into the air at Derrick, knocking him down to the ground again. Dare stood a couple of inches away from Derrick's face, barking ferociously loud, with saliva dripping into Derrick's eyes. After ten seconds of furious barking, Dare put his jaws around Derrick's throat. He was going to bite it clean off, but his master screamed out.

"No! Dare, no!" Dare kept Derrick pinned there on the ground. Derrick could feel Dare's razor sharp teeth slightly biting his throat. Derrick knew that this dog could easily kill him. So the first thing he did was to piss in his pants as he looked at Thomas and begged for mercy.

"I am sorry for what we did to you! We both give you our word! Never again will we try to steal your fish, or bother you and your dog." Dare could sense the sincerity in Derrick's voice. Thomas looked over at James, who was nodding his head in agreement with what his brother had just said.

Thomas turned to Dare, saying, "Release him." At his master's command, Dare let go of Derrick and walked over to his master, while keeping eye contact with his two foes. Foaming at the mouth, Dare continued to growl at them with his huge fangs fully exposed. Thomas patted Dare on the head while looking at Derrick saying, "I have just now saved your life by calling my dog off of you."

Derrick was still shaking with fear. He nodded his head yes, as he replied. "I do know that and thank you." After this was said, Thomas raised his voice, pointing his finger at them.

"However, I shall tell my dog to tear the faces off both of you unless you keep the oaths ye just made!"

Derrick and James both quickly responded, "We will." Thomas smiled, knowing that the problem with these two bullies was now resolved. "Alright then, ye two are free to leave. My dog will not harm ye." After Thomas said this, James and Derrick turned and ran away from there. Thomas turned to Dare, wrapping his arms around him.

"Thanks mate. I think thou didst frighten them much more than they frightened me." Thomas noticed Derrick's knife and he walked over and picked it up.

"In fact, thou hast given them such fright that they forgot this knife." Thomas did some shadow-fighting with the knife near Dare, telling him, "I will never let anyone hurt thee." Dare licked his master's other hand, the one which wasn't holding the knife, "I feel the same, master, only a hundred fold."

# CHAPTER VII
# SYMPATHY FOR THE ABUSED

Now that Dare was there, Thomas felt like fishing again. "Let us see if we can catch some more fish today," Thomas said, smiling at Dare. All of a sudden, Thomas took off running, getting a head start, while saying, "I will race you to the river. Last one there is a rotten egg." Dare followed close behind, and like always, he let his master win by just an inch. After winning, Thomas put his fishing gear down and collapsed on the ground, desperately trying to catch his breath. Dare, on the other hand, breathed normal as he licked his master on the nose. Thomas eventually caught his breath, and rose to his feet, doing a hokey little dance to celebrate his victory, while taunting Dare, pointing his finger at him with a big smile, "I am still faster than you mate, and always shall be." Dare sat there, looking up at his master with his tail wagging, turning his head sideways as if he was thinking sarcastically, "Whatever you say master, whatever you say." Thomas soon got his line out into the water again. This time, Dare was with him. Thomas did not know it, but one reason he was so successful in catching fish was because of Dare. Dare would instinctively go up stream a ways, then run, jump and splash in the water. This caused more fish to swim close to where his master was fishing. Then, Dare would come out of the water, go down stream a ways and do the same thing, causing even more fish to swim in his master's direction. After fishing for only about one hour, Dare helped Thomas catch seven more fish. "Most excellent! This is more like it," Thomas said, very pleased. "Thou dost bring me good fortune. I shall never again go fishing without thee! Our family will have plenty to eat for supper tonight." Thomas, with a huge smile, picked up the string of fish in one hand while Dare picked up the other end of the string with his mouth. The two walked towards home together, carrying the fish between them as a team.

Meanwhile, Derrick and James, with defeated expressions, had to face their father, who was drinking his spirits and was pissed off as usual. "Do not tell me! Ye pathetic bastards did not catch anything again. Is that not so?" Derrick and James kept silent while their father spewed out more slurred words. "I tell ye, rice and beans is getting very tiresome around here. I need more variety than rice and beans to go with me wine." Hearing and seeing their lazy father drunk again made both Derrick and James leave their house to get away from him for a while. However, their father came outside yelling and screaming at them, with his bottle in his hand. He followed Derrick and James as they continued trying to ignore him and walk away. Thomas and

Dare were half way home when they heard and saw Derrick and James's father scream at them.

"Ye are pathetic bastards! 'Tis no wonder thy mother left us! The two of ye art completely worthless! Do not dare to walk away from me whilst I am talking! I charge ye, come back, NOW! (But Derrick and James continued walking), Well, 'tis a fine thing. Ye two bloody bastards just keep walking, and never trouble to come home unless it be with some fish for me to enjoy with me wine!" After screaming this, Mr. Tate finished drinking his wine and threw the bottle at his sons. Luckily it just missed James's head. Mr. Tate then staggered home. Thomas and Dare continued to walk towards home. They both stopped at the same time, exchanging sympathetic glances.

"I would not wish on my worst enemy what those two lads have to live with," Thomas said, as he turned around with his dog, and walked back towards his two foes. Derrick and James were two lads whose mother had left them because of a drunken father. Mr. Tate heaped abuse on their bodies and their minds. This was why they were the way they were. Thomas and Dare approached Derrick and James, who both had their heads hung down low with tears lightly coming down their faces. Thomas held up four fish to them, "ye two," Thomas said in a friendly tone of voice. "Pray, do me a good turn and take this fish off my hands. My family cannot eat this much fish and I surely would hate to see them go to waste."

"You are a good lad." Derrick replied, raising his head a little. "I do know that you are only saying that because of what you just saw. You keep your fish. We are once again truly sorry for mistreating you and your dog."

"All is forgiven." Thomas replied. "We bear no hard feelings." Thomas moved his head, looking at Dare as he patted him. "Look ye, lads, even Dare is wagging his tail at ye. Go ahead, ye two can pet him. He has a very forgiving heart. He knows that ye two will not try to hurt me again." Derrick and James smiled weakly as they petted Dare. Thomas reached into his pocket, pulling out their knife and handed it to Derrick. "I do believe this belongs to the two of ye." Thomas held four of the fishes up to them again. "Pray reconsider and take these fish, or they shall go to waste."

Derrick closed his eyes and thought about it for a second, then opened his eyes with a half smile as he said, "We will accept your fish, if in return you accept this knife."

Thomas looked at Dare, asking, "Well, what do you think mate? Should we trade?" Dare gave a bark. Thomas gave Derrick a disappointed look, then with a great big smile, took the knife out of Derrick's extended hand as he shook it, saying "Dare says you have a bargain, mate!" In exchange, Thomas handed over four very large fish to Derrick and James.

"Our thanks, Thomas," James said, as he held the fish up to his face to smell them. "You have no idea how long it has been since we ate fish."

"My pleasure," Thomas replied.

James looked at Thomas' fishing gear and said, "I notice you do well at fishing. Have you a secret?"

Thomas opened up his little pouch, and handed James and Derrick some cheese, line and hooks. "Try this. It really works for me, especially the cheese, which is made by my mother."

"Cheese!" James replied stunned. "'Tis strange. We were told worms be the best bait."

"Worms are good bait, do not misunderstand me." Thomas replied with a slight smile. "However, this cheese is better because it floats."

"It floats?" James replied surprised. "I have never heard of that."

"Yes, 'tis true," Thomas responded nodding his head, "when it is used with the line and hooks that I just handed you." James and Derrick exchanged excited looks.

Derrick shook Thomas' hand saying, "Our thanks. We both look forward to fishing with your method tomorrow."

Thomas patted Derrick on the shoulder. "Good luck. I am sure ye lads will catch some fish. If ye like my mother's cheese, let me know and I will give ye some more."

"Thanks mate." Derrick and James both replied.

"Ye are both more than welcome." Thomas said, smiling. James looked at Dare, impressed by how he sat calmly next to his master, watching over his every move. Derrick admired the way Dare had defended his master and had been in 'kill mode' regarding himself and his brother a short while ago. But now he was nice like a little puppy, wagging his tail, knowing that he and his brother were no longer a threat to his master. This really impressed the two brothers, who told Thomas, "Dare is the best dog we have ever seen in our lives."

"My thanks for those words," Thomas replied as he wrapped his arm around Dare's thick neck. "He is me best mate." Thomas with a huge smile and Dare with his tail wagging, said their goodbyes. On their way home, Thomas patted Dare on the shoulder. "Is that not something, mate? Why, not yet an hour ago, those two were our biggest foes. Now they are our friends. I guess the good Lord really does work in mysterious ways!"

Derrick and James waited a few hours, hoping their father would sober up a little before they returned home. Upon arriving home, the brothers found their father on a cot, passed out from drinking. James covered his father with a blanket to keep him warm. Shaking their heads in disgust, the brothers walked through the house and out into the back yard. The lads prepared themselves a nice fire and cooked the fish. After they ate, James put a piece of fish and some rice on a plate for their father. The lads walked up to their father, trying to wake him up for supper, but they couldn't, so they left the fish on a small table next to their father. James wrote a little note.

"Dear father, our thanks for the good advice about befriending Thomas and asking him to advise us how to catch fish. We did as you said. We do hope you enjoy your supper. We expect to bring more fish back tomorrow for you. With love, from your two sons." James cringed and was hesitant when he wrote "with love, from your two sons." James showed these words to Derrick who also cringed. This was something that hadn't been said in years.

Right after Derrick and James left the fish and note for their father and went to bed, their father awoke. He had to take a massive piss from all the wine he had consumed. Mr.Tate didn't notice the fish and the note until he came back from the privy. He ate the fish and rice, and then passed out again.

The next morning Derrick and James got up early to go fishing. They used the lines and cheese that Thomas had given them and had great success, catching three fish each. That morning, Mr. Tate woke up with a bad headache. He read the note his sons had left. Next, he slowly got up, grabbed his bottle of wine, and walked to the privy to take another massive piss. After he walked out, he put the bottle of wine up to his mouth. Just as the wine was about to touch his lips, he stopped himself and thought about the note his sons had left, especially the part where it said "love, your sons." Mr. Tate said to himself, "How could they possibly write those words after the harsh treatment I have heaped upon them all these years?" He shook his head, walked back over to the little table, picked the note up and read that part again. Mr. Tate slowly put the bottle of wine back up to his lips and was about to take a sip but then stopped again. This time he walked outside and threw the bottle of wine against a rock. Shortly afterwards, Derrick and James came home. This time their father wasn't drinking, but was crying.

"Why so sad father?" James asked holding the fish up to him. "Look you what we brought home for you."

But his father cried all the more. "I have been nothing but a terrible father to ye two lads!" Mr. Tate said, disgusted with himself. "'Tis I myself the reason thy mother left! All I do is sit around drinking and swearing! Henceforth, I will no longer drink, but will spend more time with thee, and be a better father." He felt better about himself as he said this, knowing there was still hope for him. "Pray, wilt thou forgive me for the way I have constantly mistreated thee?" Hearing this, Derrick and James ran over to their father, giving him a great big hug.

"Of course we do forgive thee, Father," they both answered, with tears of joy trickling down their faces. Mr. Tate looked at a portrait on the wall of their mother, the woman who had been his wife, as he held his sons.

"As soon as I clean myself up, I shall go to thy mother, and beg her forgiveness. I will tell her that I am now no longer drinking and will try to win her back." Mr. Tate soon did as he said, winning his wife back. He didn't have to try to win her heart again, because she had never stopped loving him. The Tates were soon a happy family again.

# CHAPTER VIII
# THE TERROR!!

Today was Tiny's first birthday. Lord Riley walked over to Tiny's cage and took him out. "Happy birthday, Tiny. 'Tis time for thee to accomplish what I have kept thee alive for the past year to do." Lord Riley looked at Tiny skeptically. "I do surely hope thou wilt give Goliath a little bit of a challenge before he kills thee," Lord Riley said with a quiet but sinister laugh.

When Tiny entered the pit, he looked into Goliath's eyes. Tiny knew that Goliath was focused in on him in 'kill mode' and that he was going to be in a fight to the death. As soon as the fight started, Tiny's natural kill drive was born. Tiny ran circles around Goliath, as Goliath tried to bite Tiny, but was unable to. The two dogs created a cloud of dust as they ran around, so Lord Riley could not see what was going on. When the cloud of dust eventually cleared, Lord Riley looked in disbelief. With his jaw dropped to his chin, he shook his head back and forth as he mumbled, "I do not believe my eyes!" Lord Riley saw Tiny on top of Goliath, pinning him to the ground. Tiny had his jaws around Goliath's throat. "No dog has ever come close to defeating Goliath!" Lord Riley said amazed, "especially not a dog less than half his size! Lord Riley called Tiny to come. Tiny let go of Goliath, who slowly rose to his feet. His neck was bloody, and he was cowering and slinking to a corner to get away from Tiny. Tiny walked over to Lord Riley and was rewarded with a pat on his head. This was the first time in Tiny's life he had received any kind of praise. In awe, Lord Riley told him, "Thou didst exceptionally well. I need only train thee to show no mercy and to finish off thine opponents." Lord Riley whistled, twisting his neck with eyes wide open, thinking about how close he had been to leaving Tiny in the forest to die. With greed in his heart, Lord Riley said to Tiny, "'Tis a good thing I spared thy life. Thou wilt make me a lot of money!" Lord Riley watched Goliath standing at the opposite end of the pit, shaking in terror. Pleased, Lord Riley nodded his head, and looked at Tiny saying, "Henceforth, thy new name shall be Terror."

One week later, Lord Riley entered Terror in a dogfight. The people in the crowd laughed when they saw Terror about to fight Sir Gregory Lloyd's most powerful dog, a Mastiff twice Terror's size; however, three seconds into the fight, nobody was laughing, especially not Sir Gregory. For Terror quickly broke two of the Mastiff's legs, pinning the large dog to the ground by the throat, just like he had done to Goliath. After the fight, Lord Riley, was a very rich man. He had bet two hundred and fifty pounds at fifty-to-one that Terror would win. Lord Riley left the fight with twelve thousand five hundred pounds that night. On the way home, Lord Riley scolded Terror, saying "Again thou didst show mercy by not finishing off your opponent. Therefore I shall treat thee more cruelly than any creature has ever been treated, to break thee of this horrible habit!"

When Lord Riley arrived home, he counted his money and smiled as he looked at Terror saying, "I did surely earn a great deal of money today. Oh, by the way, here is thy share for helping me get so rich." Lord Riley gave Terror a whole live chicken that Terror devoured completely. During the next several weeks, Lord Riley entered Terror in more matches, making a lot more money. Lord Riley became the talk of England as having perhaps the best fighting dog in history.

# CHAPTER IX
# EVIL PLOT TO CREATE
# ULTIMATE KILLERS

Lord Riley wanted more dogs like Terror, with short snouts and wrinkled faces. So he went up to where the youngsters of the town were playing, but when they saw Lord Riley, they all ran from him. Lord Riley chased them, saying "Fear not. I come as a friend. I want only to give ye my proper thanks for what ye did for me and to pay you more money."

"Thanks, but no," the youngsters replied, as they kept running. "We picked up your dog leavings once, and that is enough." Lord Riley followed, running. He took ten pence out of his pocket, throwing the money in front of the youngsters as they ran. Charles saw the coins and stopped to pick them up. Cautiously, he turned to look back at Lord Riley, who was holding up four shillings for Charles to see.

"Pray, do not run from me any more mate." Lord Riley said gasping for air. "I only wish to ask thee some questions, for which I will gladly pay thee all this."

From a safe distance, Charles asked, "Will you pay me first?"

Without hesitation, Lord Riley responded, "Yes! And then some." Charles stopped running and Lord Riley bent over, still gasping for air. "Here are six more pence just for stopping." Lord Riley put the money on the ground, and moved ten feet away. Charles' eyes lit up seeing this, and he walked over to the money to pick it up.

"My thanks. Now what can I help you with?"

Lord Riley answered, "You know that dog I saw ye poppets with about a year ago, the dog that I called a freak of nature?" Charles slowly backed up, thinking, *Oh yes. The one we mated with your finest female, for which you wanted to kill us.* Charles thought Lord Riley still had a vendetta against him. He turned and was just about to run when Lord Riley blurted out, "Pray, do not be afraid. I do love that dog! In fact, when ye poppets arranged for that dog to mate with mine, they produced the best dog I have ever seen!"

Charles' jaw dropped when he heard this. "Are you serious?" he responded, shaking his head in disbelief.

"Yes, very much in fact." Lord Riley answered. "I will even give thee ten more pence right now if thou wilt tell me the name of that wonderful dog, and who that dog's owner is." Charles did not want to get burned by Lord Riley again, so he planned to make sure that Lord Riley paid up before he gave him any information.

Charles extended his hand, saying "'Tis a bargain." Lord Riley quickly put ten pence in Charles's hand. "That dog's name was Rascal. His owner is a lad named Thomas Gentry."

"What dost thou mean, *was*?" responded Lord Riley, in an angry tone of voice, as Charles backed up again and answered, "Unfortunately, Rascal died about nine months ago."

Lord Riley closed his eyes and took a very deep breath. Then he slapped himself on the forehead with both hands, yelling, "Damnation! I wanted to start a new breed. That dog was the key ingredient." Lord Riley continued after taking more deep breaths and calming down. "Lad, dost thou know if that dog has any littermates still alive today?"

"I most certainly do." Charles answered with a big smile on his face, and holding out his hand." Lord Riley once again put ten pence in Charles' hand, and Charles put the money in his pocket. "Indeed he does." Lord Riley was greatly relieved to hear Charles' answer. His eyes lit up again with great anticipation. He handed Charles ten more pence.

"Where can I find the littermates, and who is the owner?"

"The owner is Thomas Gentry's Uncle Robert," Charles answered. "The dog's name is Blaze. In looks, he is very like Rascal. In fact, for some strange reason, for over two hundred years, distant relatives of Thomas have continued breeding dogs that look like Rascal."

"Over two hundred years." Lord Riley responded, squinting. "That's strange, that's just like my family. How dost thou know this?"

"Because my family is very close to the Gentry family," Charles answered. "They have attended the same church for several years. My father heard this story from Thomas' uncle and he told me."

"That is a very interesting story," Lord Riley responded. "Now, canst thou tell me where Robert Gentry lives?" For a brief moment, Charles remembered how disappointed he and his friends had been when they picked up the leavings of Lord Riley's dogs. They didn't even get paid enough to buy two apple tarts. Charles knew how badly Lord Riley wanted this information, so he thought. *Now is my chance to get the money my friends and I deserve and then some, for doing Lord Riley's dirty work.*

So Charles told Lord Riley, "If you give me ten more shillings, I will take you to the house of Thomas' uncle, where Blaze lives."

"Thou hast a bargain!" Lord Riley answered with a devious smile on his face. "Now lead the way."

Charles again held out his hand. "You know what I am about to ask." Lord Riley sighed, handing Charles ten more shillings.

"Here, my lad. Thou hast better not be lying to me. Again I say, lead the way." Charles took Lord Riley to the house where Thomas' uncle lived. When they arrived, Lord Riley was greatly impressed with what he saw there, which was a lot of dogs running around, playing in the yard behind the house. Lord Riley had never seen animals able to run as fast or jump as high as these dogs. He said to himself, "'Tis no wonder Terror is so agile and quick. If I can combine the agility of these dogs with the strength of my huge dogs, I will create the best fighting dogs in history." Just then, five rabbits escaped from a small hole underneath the fence. Charles and Lord Riley both watched.

"I have seen this before." Charles said smiling. "They shall not get far."

Hearing this, Lord Riley shook his head as he replied, "That is most absurd. The rabbits have just escaped and now are free." Just when Lord Riley thought he couldn't be any more impressed, he was wrong. Charles pointed Blaze out to him.

"Look you at that white dog with dark patches over his eyes, jumping over all the other dogs, running faster than the wind. Right now he is clearing that seven foot fence and chasing all five rabbits back into the yard."

Lord Riley watched with his mouth wide open, amazed. "Ah, yes!" Charles chuckled at Lord Riley's response.

"Well, that one is Blaze." Lord Riley had just witnessed an animal move faster than anything he thought possible. When Blaze was finished herding the rabbits, he jumped back over the fence in a single bound, then he went over to the hole that the rabbits had used to escape, and filled it back up with his front paws. Afterwards, Blaze went back to his little doghouse and went back to sleep as if nothing had happen. Lord Riley shook his head in awe, his mouth still open.

"I must possess that dog!" Lord Riley said with a selfish vision. "Charles, if thou dost go along with what I say, and I can persuade Robert to sell me that fine dog, I shall give thee an extra eight shillings as a bonus."

"Good, the money would be welcome." Charles replied, unenthusiastic. "'Tis unfortunate but I do not think Thomas' uncle can be persuaded to sell Blaze at any price." As Charles knocked on the door of Thomas uncles' house, Lord Riley patted him on the shoulder.

"Oh ye of little faith! Never underestimate the power of money. Watch and learn, lad!" Lord Riley said arrogantly. Robert opened the door. A huge smile filled his face as soon as he saw Charles.

"My, what a pleasing surprise! How goes it with thee and with thy parents?" Robert asked as he shook Charles' hand.

"My parents and I are quite well," Charles answered. "My thanks. How goes it with you, Mr. Gentry?"

"Oh busy as I always am, Charles, fishing or tending to my farm, but that's the way I love life. Blaze and I went fishing today and caught a lot of fish. Here are some for thee to take home to your parents." Charles took a string of five fish from Robert, who was very pleased.

"My thanks for your kindness. I am sure my family will enjoy the fish." Robert got an eerie feeling about Lord Riley. He glanced at him with slightly narrowed eyes.

"Who's your friend, Charles? He looks familiar." Before Charles could introduce him, Lord Riley extended his hand and introduced himself with a phony smile.

"I am Lord Riley Braun Warne. It is indeed a pleasure to meet you!" Lord Riley paused in awe, thinking about Blaze, before going on. "I must say, Robert, the good Lord sure blessed you with some very impressive looking dogs. I do believe you must have some interesting stories to tell about them, which I would love to hear." Hearing this, Robert's eyes, which had been slightly narrowed with suspicion, opened wide as he smiled broadly. The two things Robert loved more than anything were his dogs and God. Robert had never had any children, so his dogs were like children to him. The best way to break the ice with Robert, and make friends with him, was to exalt God, and to show an interest in his dogs. Lord Riley knew this, and that is exactly what he did.

Robert, still smiling from hearing his dogs praised as a divine blessing, said "Well, ye two, do not just stand there; pray, enter and join me for some tea."

"My thanks. I would be delighted," Lord Riley replied as he followed Charles into the house. "I do declare, Robert, your home is most impressive. It reminds me of my place, with the dogs roaming all around, happy and free, like they own the place. Yes I say, just like my place!"

"That makes me very happy, knowing your dogs also have a good home." Robert replied as he poured tea. "I would like to come over some time and see them."

"Pray, do. You and your dogs would be most welcome guests at any time!" replied Lord Riley with a gulp, knowing full well that Robert would never speak to him again if he were to come over and see how he abused his dogs. However, with his phony smile, Lord Riley went on to say, "Charles has visited my home several times to play with my dogs and always has a good time." Hearing this, Charles rolled his eyes, knowing that Lord Riley had just flatly lied. Picking up dog leavings for no money is hardly a good time. Nor were Lord Riley's dogs happy and free, but were always miserable and chained up, except when their time had come to be thrown into a pit to fight a dog or a bull to the death. Ignorant of all of this, Robert smiled along with Lord Riley and handed him a cup of tea.

"My thanks," Lord Riley replied, taking the tea from Robert's hand

"'Tis My pleasure," Robert answered with a smile, knowing Lord Riley would love his tea. "'Tis surely good to know that there are people in the world like you and me who treat man's best friend with love and respect." Lord Riley nodded his head in apparent agreement with Robert.

"I do agree! I do surely wish there were more people who treated man's best friend in this manner. 'Tis shameful that so many cruel people who own dogs mistreat and abuse them." After saying this, Lord Riley took a sip of Robert's tea. As soon as he swallowed it, Lord Riley's eyes lit up.

"Astounding! This is the best tasting tea I have ever had in my life!"

Robert wasn't surprised to hear this. He replied, "I have been told that from time to time." Just about everything that Lord Riley had told Robert was a lie, but he was serious about the tea.

Lord Riley then assumed a very sad look, saying, "'Tis not right to think thus, being the God fearing person that I am, but sometimes I do wish that God would take vengeance and make all those dog abusers suffer the way they cause man's best friends to suffer!"

Robert nodded his head in agreement with Lord Riley and replied, "Oh no, do not feel bad for thinking that way, brother. Sometimes I do feel the same way myself." Charles, with both hands on his face, lifted his head up and shook it back and forth, thinking, *"I have never heard anybody in my life tell more lies and look so convincing while telling them."* Seeing his reaction, Lord Riley stood directly in front of Charles to block Robert's view of him. Lord Riley knew that if Robert saw Charles' reaction, he wouldn't believe in his lies.

Lord Riley, very intrigued with the drawings of dogs on Robert's walls, commented, "I see that you have some fine art works. Would these be drawings of your dogs?"

Robert answered, "Some are, and some were owned by my ancestors and have been passed down from generation to generation to me. When I die, all these paintings shall be given to my favorite nephew, Thomas." Robert focused his attention on Charles. "By the way, how goes it with my favorite nephew?"

"I do believe Thomas is doing very well," answered Charles. "When Rascal died, I thought Thomas would fall apart. However, every time I see Thomas, he has a big smile on his face and the dog that he found in the forest is always by his side. I think God put that dog there to help heal Thomas' broken heart." Hearing this made Robert feel very good.

"Thou art a smart lad, Charles. I think God's help kept that young dog alive in the forest so that the dog and my nephew would find each other. The good Lord works in mysterious ways!" Robert shook his head in awe, thinking about Dare, as he went on to say, "Never have I seen a better dog for herding cows than Dare. He is both quick and agile like my dogs, but with the strength of a bull. I would not have believed it possible for a dog to be better at herding than one of my dogs."

Robert suddenly hung his head low, thinking of a painful experience in the past. "My nephew is like me. I can remember the pain I felt when I lost my first dog at his age. Two things that helped heal my broken heart were God and another dog." Lord Riley didn't believe in God or like hearing about Him. As far as he was concerned, he himself was God. Lord Riley knew that Dare had been put in the forest by himself, not by God. But Lord Riley was astonished to hear that his favorite dog had a brother that was both alive and well. He thought for sure that there was no way that any of the dogs left out in that cold forest would have survived on their own.

Intrigued, Lord Riley asked Robert, "Pray tell, did your nephew find any more dogs out there?" Robert hung his head low again as he answered.

"I asked my nephew that same question and my nephew started to cry. So I hugged him, knowing the answer to my question." Lord Riley thought, *"Oh pray spare me this pitiful drama! And to think it is over some stupid dogs! I do not give a bloody rat's ass about any dog's feelings! I just care about how much money I can make from fighting dogs in the pit, killing bulls and other dogs, and from breeding them."* After thinking this, Lord Riley looked at Robert with a phony, sad look.

"It breaks my heart to hear of such a catastrophe. I hope the good Lord strikes with lightening the wicked soul who abandoned those dogs in the forest." Charles, hearing Lord Riley say this, took a few steps away from him. Robert took another sip of tea, raising his head high.

"Let us talk about something more pleasant. Charles, does my nephew ever play with thee and the youngsters of the town?"

"No, not really," Charles answered. "I do not talk to Thomas very much. He and I greet each other, and perhaps talk for a minute or two every now and then. But Thomas keeps mainly to himself and does everything with his dog." A look of conviction suddenly came upon Charles as he continued talking. "I do think this is because he really loves his dog and some of me friends mocked him about how funny his dog looks. 'Tis a pity, but I do think this really hurt his feelings."

"That sounds much like myself when I was his age," Robert replied with a slight chuckle, "because my dog looked so different from any other dog, with his wrinkled skin and short muzzle. I was also mocked and was extremely sensitive about my dog, not wanting to have anything to do with anyone who made fun of my dog. Do be patient Charles, give Thomas time and continue to be nice to him. Just like me, he shall soon grow up and not be so sensitive about what people say." Robert smiled, pausing, taking another sip of tea. "I do declare, 'twas very strange that the youngsters who ridiculed my dogs most strongly were the first to buy puppies from me when we got older, and from the same line of dogs as those they had mocked, for they remembered the great skill of my dogs at herding livestock. Once they had owned one of my dogs, they never considered purchasing a dog from anyone else."

"Indeed, I noticed when I walked up here." Lord Riley sincerely replied. "The working ability of your dogs is very impressive. Judging by the dogs in your yard and these drawings of your dogs from the past, I do not see how anyone could make fun of such appealing and unusual looking dogs." Hearing this, Robert gave a slight chuckle, unaware that Lord Riley had seen one of his dogs before.

"Many thanks! You are the first person outside my family to ever say that upon seeing my dogs for the first time."

While Robert said this, Lord Riley had a moment of deja vu as he saw a picture of a dog that looked extremely familiar. Lord Riley put his tea down got up out of his chair, and walked up close to the picture and said with a bedazzled look, "I know that I have seen this dog somewhere before! Pray tell me about him."

Robert chuckled as he answered. "'Tis impossible, unless you were alive about three hundred years ago! That dog was found October 30th, 1211, by one of my distant ancestors by the name of Byron Gentry, just outside the town of Stamford. That dog's name was Noble. Byron wrote that the Heavens arranged that he should meet Noble. Noble saved his livestock from disaster several times. Byron wrote that Noble's love for him was the only thing that healed him and kept him from dying from a broken heart, which he had suffered at the tragic loss of Marilyn, his beloved wife. Noble was the first working dog in the Gentry family, and was the foundation sire for dogs in the Gentry family. He has been carefully line bred by my relatives over the centuries. Noble's bloodlines and spirit are very strong in my dogs today. His bloodlines will remain in my dogs for future generations to come." Lord Riley also had a lot of drawings of the dogs of distant relatives in his family. Hearing this story and seeing a drawing of Noble influenced Lord Riley to suddenly have a strong memory of a piece of art that he had received from a distant relative, entitled The One That Got Away, by William Warne. William had drawn a picture of a dog that looked very similar to Noble. William also wrote a poem, in line with this art piece, entitled the one that got away which went:

In The Wee houre, Thou Layeste a'sleape
Uponne Thy Floore. Soone a'wakenned
Bye a Loude Uproare, To The Sounde
Of howlynge Thou Canst Not Ignorre.
Leeping to Thy Feete, Thou dost Go
Toward's Thy Doore.

Outside Tis Slyte, a'Mistedde Nyghte,
But Wythe Ayde fromme Lunarr Lyghte,
Who Doth Shyne e'er so Bryghte,
Thou Canst see Everrie Thyng In
Syghte.

At Fyrste, Thou Dost Not Beeleeve
What eyes Conceeve.

Fore Out of The Fogge, a'peeres a
Ghoste seem'd Dogge,
Followe'd bye His Packe, Soone They
Engayge Ande Attacke,

A Large Bulle, that Shalle Mayke
Them Fulle.

Thyne Towne's biggeste Fears
Reappeer,
The Hounds of Hell Relees'd From
Theyr cell.

Cravynge Bloode that Is Freshe,
They rippe at The Fleshe.

But Woe, Deathe commes Firste,
Packe Leaderre's Friende Dealte
Worste. Throughe His eyes,
He doth witnesse Frieyndes Demyse.

Scorn'd fromme the horne,
As Fleshe Was Torne.

Leaderres' Will, Longynge To Kille.

Wythe a Tenayciousse Gryppe,
He Goes for Foes noes, Untylle
Tis ripp'd, And All Bloode Flowes.

Leaderre of Packe hath Revpeynge
Backe, Fore Deathe of They Frende,
As Bulles' Lyfe commeth to An Ende.

That Nyghte I look'd Throughe a Walle.
Wytnes'd Dogs Smalle ande Talle,
Admyrynge alle.

Especiallie the One Who Coulde run,
Seconde To None,
Destroying a Bulle oberre a tonne.

Fore It Was Bye He, That Inspyr'd
Me to Creayte, Bye Fayte,
Moste Legendayrie Sporte,
Bulle Bayte.

After this memory came to Lord Riley, he sat back down in his chair
with his eyes wide open. His jaw dropped slightly, as he shook his head
back and forth in disbelief.

"How goes it with you? Are you unwell?" Robert asked, seeing Lord
Riley's traumatized expression. "You look like you've just seen a ghost."
Lord Riley didn't respond. He was too much in a daze, thinking, *What a
coincidence! The dog that my distant relative, the legendary Earl, looked
for so long and so hard was probably living no more than twenty miles away
and working on a farm. The Earl would have loved to breed to this dog and
use him and his offspring for bull baiting!*" Coming out of his trance, Lord
Riley stuttered, "Ah- excuse me- what was your question?" Robert laughed
as he asked again.

"I asked, how goes it with you? You look like you have just seen a ghost! If you did, it wouldn't surprise me because nearby in the town of Stamford, several people have claimed to have heard and seen ghosts."

Lord Riley thought. *"'Tis exactly what I was thinking!"* However, he replied as he rose to his feet, "I am fine; Just now I thought about something that happened a while ago."

# CHAPTER X
# DOGS SENSE WHAT MAN CANNOT

Lord Riley reached into his pockets and pulled out all the money he had, which was a large amount. He put it all into Robert's hand, then turned and looked out at Blaze in Robert's yard. "Robert, me mate," Lord Riley said with confidence, "I do love your dog Blaze. In fact, I want to own him! I have just handed you enough money to go out and buy a hundred dogs. However, for some reason, if you do not think that is money enough, I will gladly give you more."

Robert looked at the money he was holding in his hand, and whistled, "Ye gods! 'Tis indeed a lot of money. 'Tis true, it could buy a hundred dogs!" Robert didn't think twice as he handed the money back to Lord Riley. "However, it can not buy Blaze! I am sorry, but Blaze is not for sale at any price. He is like a son to me." Lord Riley saw the strong sincere look and love Robert had for Blaze in his eyes. He knew that even if he offered Robert all the money in the world, it would just be a waste of breath.

Lord Riley smiled, patting Robert on the shoulder. "You are a man after my own heart. I would do exactly the same were I offered this amount of money for one of my favorite dogs." Lord Riley took Robert's hand and put the money back in it. "Pray keep this money in exchange for first pick of Blaze's next litter, and allow me to use Blaze for stud service on some of me bitches."

"I do believe we can arrange that, " Robert replied with a smile. "In fact, right now Blaze and my favorite female dog, Sly Ann, have a litter of ten pups that are seven weeks old. However, whenever I sell a pup to someone, they first have to pass a little test." Lord Riley kept smiling as he thought, *"What a moron. He knows I will pay him more money than any one else will! And he is going to give me a test!"*

However, Lord Riley replied, "I will gladly take your test. What is it that you want me to do?"

"You do not do a thing." Robert answered, "Before I ever sell a pup to someone, I always have the mother of the puppies look over and smell the person. If she accepts you, then you can have one of her puppies. If she doesn't, well I hope there will be no hard feelings between us."

"You do not have to worry about Sly Ann not liking me," replied Lord Riley confident Sly Ann couldn't see the evil that lurked within him. "I have never in me life met a dog that I did not love or that did not loved me back. I do respect you, though, for making sure that your puppies go to good homes.

My home for instance, is a place where your pup will be loved and cared for and treated like royalty. I can not wait to meet Sly Ann." Lord Riley told a bunch of lies, but this was the biggest lie of all.

Hearing this, Robert rose from his chair, walked to the back door and opened it, saying, "Well, there is no better time than the present." Robert whistled, "Come here, Sly Ann!" Sly Ann instantly came running into the house.

Robert pointed at Lord Riley, who was down on all fours making ridiculous goo, goo, ga ga, baby faces at her while complimenting Sly Ann, saying "What a beautiful fawn dog. I especially like her unique, darkly lined eyes. Come here, pretty girl."

Sly Ann looked at Robert who looked back, asking, "Well now, Sly Anne. Thou dost know the routine. What dost thou think?" Sly Ann walked towards Lord Riley, staring deep into his eyes. Suddenly she stopped, taking in a few deep breaths. Her hair quickly rose on her back as she barked violently at Lord Riley. It was almost as if she could smell and sense all the blood of innocent dogs, that had been shed because of this evil man. Sly Ann's maternal instincts told her that Lord Riley would be a terrible owner for her pups. Disappointed, Robert shook his head, got down on one knee calmly petting Sly Ann on the head.

"Tis all right," he told her. "Do not fear, I shall listen to thee, just as I have always done." When Sly Ann had calmed down, Robert rose to his feet and put her back outside. He walked over to Lord Riley, handing back all his money while saying, "I am sorry that we can not do business together. I hope there are no hard feelings between us." Lord Riley clenched his fists in an effort to stay calm and not explode.

"Oh, no!" He replied with a ridiculous phony smile on his face. "No hard feelings whatsoever. However, I do not understand. This is the first time in my life that a dog did not like me and that I've been snarled at! Pray test me on another of your dogs. Perhaps Blaze? I warrant he would not bark or growl at me. After all, 'tis a lot of money that I am offering you for one of Blaze's puppies!"

Without hesitation, Robert answered, "Pray, understand me. When it comes to my dogs, money is not an issue. Sly Ann's decision is final. I am sorry but you will have to buy a dog from someone else." Hearing this, Lord Riley became enraged and could no longer control his emotions.

"I cannot believe this!" he yelled, " You are saying no to buckets of money because your stupid bitch does not like me! You, sir, have just turned down more money than anyone has ever been offered for a dog! You, sir, are the most pathetic person I have ever met in my life!" Hearing Lord Riley yelling at their master, the dogs all ran to the back door, barking violently and clawing at the door, trying to get in to make Lord Riley fully aware that his attitude towards their master was unacceptable. The exception was Blaze, who was the only dog able to jump up and get into the house through an eleven-foot window. Once inside, Blaze got between Lord Riley and his master. He barked at Lord Riley as if to say, "I will fight to the death if you even think about hurting my master!"

Robert walked over to the front door, opened it and said to Lord Riley, "'Tis time for you to leave." Lord Riley didn't say another word, but gave Robert and Charles looks of fury as he left the house. Charles had been thinking that perhaps Lord Riley had turned over a new leaf. However, having heard all of Lord Riley's ridiculous lies, Charles knew he had not changed. Lord Riley was just pretending to be nice, trying to get something that he really wanted for his own financial gain.

# CHAPTER XI
# STEALING CANDY FROM A BABY

Charles was glad that Robert didn't sell a puppy to Lord Riley. Even though Charles didn't get any more money from Lord Riley, he was still glad because he knew Lord Riley would have abused Robert's dogs. Charles apologized to Robert for bringing Lord Riley over.

Robert patted Charles on the shoulder, responding, "'Tis alright. Be not be severe with yourself, lad. 'Twas very hard to tell that Lord Riley is a cruel man, especially judging by his behavior. I could not tell either. That is why I always have the potential new owner looked over by the mother of the litter. In the wild, the lives of the pups depend on the instincts of their mother."

Charles took a few more sips of tea while listening, then asked, "Hast ever seen a mother dog more upset with someone than Sly Ann was at Lord Riley?"

Robert sighed, rolling his eyes as he answered, "Never like that, Charles! Never like that!"

Charles finished drinking his final sip of tea, then commented, "Until I witnessed what happened here today, I did not know how special your dogs are! As soon as I return home, I shall ask my father if I may own one of Blaze and Sly Ann's pups." Robert smiled hearing this. He opened the back door, letting Sly Ann in again and pointed at Charles.

"Well Sly Ann, once again thou dost know our custom. What think ye of this one?" Sly Ann stared in Charles eyes as she slowly walked up to him. She walked around him, sniffing him up and down. Afterwards, with her mouth she grabbed a towel that was on the floor and invited Charles to grab the other end. The two played tug of war for the next several minutes. When they were finished playing, Sly Ann licked Charles on his hand and walked away with her tail wagging. Seeing this, Robert put his hand back on Charles' shoulder. With a big smile, Robert opened the back door and walked out with Charles and Sly Ann. As soon as they took two steps into the back yard, Sly Ann's puppies came running over to meet and greet them.

"Tis all right," Robert told Charles. "Take your pick. Whatever dog thou dost desire is thine."

Charles turned away from the puppies saying, "I must not become too attached to them, in case my father says no."

Robert chuckled as he responded, "I do assure thee, there is no need to fret about that! Every time thy father has been here, he tells me how much he loves my dogs. He also told me, 'if ever my son wanted a dog, you would be the person from whom I would purchase a dog'. So, if thou dost still desire to have one of these pups, thou canst have one at no cost. Go ahead!" Robert said while picking up a couple of the pups. "Take thy pick. Which pup will be the lucky new owner of thee?" Charles smiled as he rolled around the ground, laughing and playing with the pups.

"That is the best news ever I have heard in my life." Charles said as he rose to his feet and gave Robert a great big hug. Charles picked up the first puppy that came to him, giving the puppy a great big kiss on the lips. "I shall take this one and shall name him Sly, because he has the same sly look in his eye that his mother has." Charles pulled out the money in his pocket saying, "I do wish to pay you."

Robert shook his head no as he responded, "I shall not hear of such nonsense. Thy new pup is a gift from me to thee. Keep thy money."

Charles shook Robert's hand. "Many thanks. I cannot say how happy you have made me."

"Thou hast made me happy, too," Robert replied, as he walked Charles and Sly to the front door, and gave Sly a goodbye kiss. "Ye two take good care of each other. I am certain that the two of ye will be the best of friends. Please return for a visit anytime ye wish."

"Again, my thanks," Charles replied, "We will."

Hearing this, Robert smiled, saying, "We are glad to hear that." Sly Ann was next to Robert on the front porch, wagging her tail. Charles thanked Robert again for everything, then turned and walked away. He took about one hundred steps before turning around and saw Robert and Sly Ann both waving goodbye. Charles waved back as he continued walking home.

When Charles was about a quarter of the way home he ran into Lord Riley, who was waiting for him.

"Oh, splendid. I see that thou hast gotten yourself a pup!" Lord Riley said with a big sinister smile on his face. "I would have asked that thou obtain a pup for me from that obsessed dog loving fool. However I see that thou hast already done so. Thou shalt be paid eight more shillings for that pup."

Charles put his hand up. "My thanks, but no! My pup is not for sale!"

Hearing this, Lord Riley walked towards Charles with the money in his hand saying, "Look thou, my lad, give me little Rover and receive your money; otherwise your life may be over!" Charles held Sly close to his chest with both arms as he backed away from him.

"I said no! I will not sell me new mate to you at any price!"

"Thou art the smartest, most loyal of lads ever I have met in my life." Lord Riley commended him. "Therefore, I shall pay thee sixteen shillings to return to Robert's residence and fetch me the fastest male pup he has.

Tell Robert that thou dost want a companion and playmate for thy new pup." Charles glanced at the sixteen shillings in Lord Riley's hand.

Without hesitation, Charles answered, "My thanks, but no, milord." Lord Riley closed his eyes while taking a deep breath and commended Charles again.

"Thou art a smarter lad than I thought. So be it. I shall pay thee one pound and eight shillings for a pup of Robert's."

Again Charles responded with, "Again, my thanks, but no, milord." Now, Lord Riley was starting to get very angry. He began to raise his voice and wave his hands close to Charles.

"Alright, lad! Thou dost win! I shall give thee three pounds for the dog in thine hands! 'Tis my final offer! What say thee now?" Charles became frightened because Lord Riley raised his hands and voice out of anger and frustration.

With his puppy securely close to his chest, Charles firmly answered, "NO! All your money cannot compare to the love I have for my new pup! I, like Robert Gentry, shall not sell him at any price. Now, pray leave us in peace!" Charles turned with Sly in his arms and ran away.

As Lord Riley watched Charles run away, he shook his head and mumbled, "What a fool! I do not intend to let that pup get away from me!" Lord Riley ran after Charles, chasing him through small streams and over hills for a couple of miles. Just when Lord Riley was about to completely run out of breath, he finally caught Charles, grabbing his left arm.

Charles screamed, "HELP!"

But Lord Riley just laughed and said, "Go ahead and scream your lungs out, thou stupid lad! Thou art wasting thy breath, for nobody is around to hear thee scream." Lord Riley then grabbed Charles by the ankles and flipped the boy over, lifting both Charles and Sly in the air and causing all of Charles's money to drop to the ground. Lord Riley was wrong when he told Charles that nobody was around to hear him scream, because Thomas and Dare were playing fetch the stick not too far away. As soon as Charles yelled for help, Dare heard him. With the stick in his mouth, Dare raised his head and moved it from side to side, listening carefully to determine the direction from which Charles's screams were coming. Once Dare had pinpointed the direction, he froze for a second, dropping his stick and turned towards Thomas. But instead of giving his master a normal, friendly, playful bark, Dare gave a deep warning bark that meant something was wrong. Dare turned in the direction of the sound of yelling, and started running towards Charles. Thomas knew that Dare was greatly troubled about something and wanted him to follow, so Thomas ran as fast as he possibly could behind Dare. Meanwhile, Lord Riley carried Charles and Sly to a nearby cliff, and held both of them over the edge, threatening, "Unless thou dost instantly hand over that pup in your arms, ye shall both be splattered against the rocks."

Screaming at the top of his lungs, Charles responded, "Alright! You win! Pray, have mercy!"

Hearing this, Lord Riley arrogantly replied, "Ha!" then pulled Charles and Sly away from the cliff while warning Charles, "Put down my new pup, or I shall put ye two back over the cliff. Next time, I shall let go of thee." Charles had no choice but to comply, with tears falling down and dripping off of his arms onto the ground.

Charles kissed Sly on the head, telling him, "I love thee," as he gently put Sly on the ground. After this was done, Lord Riley let Charles go. Charles broke his fall with his hands, landing safely on the ground. Sly immediately pounced on Charles, licking his face as he lay there.

Now just at that moment, Thomas and Dare showed up. Thomas put his finger to his lips, telling Dare, "Keep quiet," and they remained hidden, listening and watching from behind some bushes. Shaking his head, Lord Riley looked at Sly licking Charles's tears.

"What a pitiful sight! Well, say your final goodbyes, because after today, ye two shall never see each other again!" After a minute of Charles and Sly kissing each other, Lord Riley pulled Sly away from Charles. Sly began to cry.

Lord Riley held Sly with both hands near his face saying, "Ah, be quiet! Fighting dogs do not cry!" Lord Riley then picked up all the money that had fallen out of Charles' pockets, and turned to shake his head at him. "Foolish, foolish lad! Thou didst have the chance to make a lot of money, but instead of taking up the opportunity like any normal person would, thou didst chose a dog over money. Now thou dost have neither! What a great fool thou art!" With tears running down his face, Charles picked up a big rock.

"Put my pup down, you bloody bastard!" He yelled, "else I shall throw this at you!"

Lord Riley laughed, saying, "If thou doest, 'twill be the biggest mistake of thy short life!"

Charles lightly hit himself in the head with the hand that was holding the rock, as a couple of his tears trickled onto the rock. He looked at Sly, apologizing as he dropped the rock to the ground, afraid of accidentally hitting Sly instead of Lord Riley.

As soon as the rock hit the ground, Lord Riley chuckled, turned and started to walk away, saying, "I knew thou art a coward. Now, there is nothing to prevent me from creating more ultimate killers!"

Immediately after hearing this, Thomas, slapped Dare on the shoulder. "Well, mate! You know what to do!" Dare instantly came out from behind the bushes, circling around Lord Riley and barking ferociously. Dare stood face to face with Lord Riley, staring him right in the eyes with his massive fangs bulging out of his mouth, dripping massive amounts of saliva. Lord Riley knew that the best thing to do in this situation was to stay as still as a board. Lord Riley did this very well, except for the urine that was trickling to the ground from his shorts. He was terrified. His thoughts were, *"At any second, this fast, muscular dog, that strongly resembles my best fighting dog Terror, is going to tear me apart."* A few seconds later, which seemed like eternity to Lord Riley, Thomas came out from behind the bushes. He walked up to Dare and patted him on the head.

"Good dog!"

With a bad attitude and harsh tone of voice, Lord Riley demanded, "Order your mad beast away from me at once!"

With his eyes narrowed with anger, Thomas responded, "That so called mad beast happens to be me best mate, and mates do not order each other around. My dog has a damn good reason for wanting to attack you."

Lord Riley responded with slowly raised hands. "No, he does not!"

Enraged, Thomas picked up a rock and threw it just over Lord Riley's head. "If you do not hand over that pup in your hands to the rightful owner immediately" Thomas stressed, "Me best mate will remove your head from your body!" Hearing this, Lord Riley made his tone of voice more peaceful, and put on an innocent face. With his baby blue eyes, he attempted to play the victim.

"Why, I am the owner of this cute little puppy," he pleaded. "This lad came

to my home and tried to steal him from my garden! Fortunately, though, I came home just as he was leaving. I chased him all the way out here before finally catching him. So seest thou, I am therefore merely taking my pup, which rightfully belongs to me!" Hearing this, Dare barked even louder.

"Me mate and I know you are lying," Thomas replied, shaking his head in disgust. "For we stayed hidden, watching what you did. I do know that the pup you hold there was bred by my Uncle Robert. Never would he sell a dog to an evil doer such as yourself!" Fed up with lies, Thomas warned him again with a raging voice. "This will be the last time I say it. Hand the pup over to the rightful owner!" Lord Riley looked at Dare, who was now crouched down and ready to attack. Slowly, Lord Riley handed Sly over to Charles. Sly stopped crying as soon as Charles touched him. Charles pulled Sly close to his chest, giving him a little kiss on the head, as a tear of joy dripped down Sly's face. Seeing this, Thomas gave a quick smile at the boy and his dog, then turned back to Lord Riley and said with a frown, "The nerve of you, trying to steal a pup from a defenseless lad. I should let my dog have at you."

As Thomas said this, Dare continued to bark at Lord Riley, who replied, "Look you, I did give over the pup to the lad. Pray now tell your dog to leave me alone."

Thomas patted Dare on the head again, and smiled as he said, "We believe you are forgetting something."

Lord Riley baffled, held his hands opened and asked, "What?"

Thomas answered, "My dog will not leave you alone unless you return to Charles all the money that you took from him." Lord Riley started walking slowly backwards as Dare was making little air bites close to Lord Riley's groin area.

"But this money is . . ." but before Lord Riley could say the word mine, Dare knocked him to the ground and got right in Lord Riley's face, his fangs scraping Lord Riley's neck area.

Thomas told Lord Riley, "We are starting to tire of your lies! Now hand the money over to the rightful owner!" Lord Riley, terrified of Dare, reached in his pocket, pulling out a lot of money, and dropped it on the ground. This was even more than the amount that he originally gave to Charles.

"ALRIGHT!" Lord Riley shouted, "Here's the lad's money. Now, pray call off your beast!"

Thomas walked over to the money that Lord Riley had spilled on the ground, and picked it up with big bulging eyes, and said, "Amazing! 'Tis a lot of money, 'tis certain!" He walked over to Charles. "I do believe this is yours," Thomas said, as he handed Charles all the money.

"My thanks." Charles gratefully replied. At this moment, Lord Riley was slowly backing up, and keeping an eye on Dare with great fear. Lord Riley knew that if he moved too fast, Dare would attack.

Charles told Lord Riley, "You have given me ten shillings more than you originally gave to me!" Charles tried to return the extra money. "Look you, sir, here is the extra money. You are welcome to come and get it." However, Lord Riley continued to back up slowly, staying focused on Dare, who was staring in Lord Riley's eyes and growling quietly, looking as if he could attack at any second.

"Therefore," Lord Riley said in a gentle soft tone of voice, "You may keep it all."

"My thanks, milord!" Charles responded excitingly. "Are you certain?"

"Oh yes, quite certain, 'tis all yours," Lord Riley answered with a touch of sarcasm as he continued to slowly squirm away. When Lord Riley was a hundred feet away, Dare took his eyes off of him and walked towards Thomas and Charles. As Dare did this, Lord Riley didn't waste any time getting out of there, but turned and ran away as fast as he could. Charles turned towards Thomas, shaking his hand as he patted Dare on the head. Charles thanked both Thomas and Dare for helping him and his new friend Sly. Charles tried to give Thomas the extra ten shillings that Lord Riley had left. But Thomas absolutely refused to take any of it, no matter how hard Charles tried.

Thomas looked at Charles's puppy with a great big smile on his face saying with a grin, "Look thou, mate, that is a beautiful little pup, 'tis certain. I wonder where thou didst get him," knowing quite well that it was from his Uncle Robert.

Charles chuckled, "Methinks know where I got him. Wouldst thou like to hold him?"

Thomas held out his arms, answering, "my thanks," as he took Sly from Charles's hands and kissed Sly on top of the head. Then he held Sly out close to Dare, who gave the young pup a bath with his tongue. After Sly's bath, Thomas held Sly close to his chest and dried him off with his shirt, commenting, "Your pup is a precious thing. I am certainly glad we were here to save him from that evil Lord Riley."

Charles nodded his head in agreement, "Yes, I am glad, too."

As they were walking towards town together, Thomas said, "I am pleasantly surprised. I did not think that thou didst have much enthusiasm for my uncle's dogs."

"'Tis true," Charles replied with a slightly guilty tone, "that is, until today. For earlier, while at thine uncle's home, I saw the pups do some truly amazing things that influenced me to want one. Your uncle was quite kind, and gave me the one that thou dost carry." A guilty look suddenly came over Charles' face as his tone became even guiltier. "I do believe the reason that thou didst think I was not enthusiastic about thine uncle's dogs was that when all the town youngsters, especially Todd Everson, made their fun, I laughed right along with them, instead of defending thee and thy dogs. However, I never did dislike thy dogs." Then Charles, with his head held down, extended his hand to Thomas. "I pray thee, accept my sincere apology and be me mate."

"Certainly! I would like nothing better," Thomas answered, shaking Charles' hand.

# CHAPTER XII
# THE OUTCAST GAINS RESPECT

Shortly thereafter, they heard the voice of Todd Everson. "Well, well, what do we have here? Why 'tis Thomas Gentry, with the world's ugliest dog. Look ye, he carries an ugly pup, soon to become the future's ugliest dog." Thomas and Charles looked to their right side, only to see Todd and the rest of the youngsters of the town laughing and pointing fingers at Dare and Sly, and making other derogatory comments like, "Who punched your dogs' faces in?" and then laughing hysterically. Todd looked at Charles. "Hey mate, why art thou with them? Do not tell me that thou hast become a freak lover, too."

Charles gave Sly a pat on the head and walked over to Todd, this time sticking up for Thomas with an angry voice, "That so called future's ugliest dog, happens to be me beloved new pup! I advise thee to apologize to me mate and his dog!"

"And if I do not?" Todd responded, chuckling.

"'Twill be your face punched in, then!" Charles answered, poking Todd in the chest with his index finder.

With a cocky look on his face, Todd pushed Charles, replying, "Oh, is that so?" Todd tried to push Charles again, but this time Charles used his wrists to knock Todd's arms out of the way, then with both hands, grabbed Todd by the back of the neck and pulled Todd's face into his knee. As Todd's head snapped back, Charles punched him as hard as he could right on the jaw, knocking Todd out momentarily.

After this, Charles asked sarcastically, "Does anybody else have any compliments they care to express about these dogs?" (With fearful looks, the youngsters shook their heads no, except for Emily Sinclair, who was the first to speak up).

"Yes, I do," she said as she turned her beautiful blue eyes towards Thomas and looked him right in the eyes as she walked towards him. "I am sorry for laughing at your dogs. I shall never do so again." Emily gave Sly a kiss on the side of his cheek as she petted Dare, who wiggled his tail. Emily's sister Sara apologized likewise, followed by the rest of the town youngsters.

While this was going on, Charles stood leaning over Todd, who was still on the ground. "I demand that thou dost apologize to Thomas for thy cruel remarks!" In a daze, with a bloody nose and mouth, Todd lay still for a moment.

Turning his head toward the spot where Thomas and the dogs were standing he said, "Alright, I do apologize for my cruel remarks. Pray, forgive me." Charles looked at Thomas, who nodded his head in approval. Charles then helped Todd up with an extended hand, asking, "Art thou still me mate?"

Todd shook Charles' hand and as he was helped to his feet, answered, "Yes, of course I am!" Todd looked down at the ground and seeing some of his blood, said, "I guess I deserved that."

Charles nodded his head in agreement. "Aye, that thou didst," Charles said as he walked over to Thomas, taking the moneybag that he had received from Lord Riley. He walked back to Todd and handed him two shillings and six pence. "Thou dost also deserve this!"

Pleasantly surprised, Todd took the money asking, "What is this for?" Charles answered with a smile on his face.

"Let us just say that Lord Riley had a change of heart about paying us a pittance for picking up his dogs' leavings. The money that I just handed to you is payment for thy share of the work." Charles told the rest of the youngsters to form a line and then he handed them each two shillings and six pence. This was enough money for each of them to buy apple tarts every day for over a month. When Charles had finished paying all his friends, Emily and Sara asked Charles if they could hold his puppy. Charles didn't hesitate because he had a strong crush on Sara, and instantly handed Sly over to her.

"Gracious! What an adorable pup," Sara said, "I especially like his sweet little wrinkles."

Emily sighed and looked at Sly, commenting, "We would love to have a pup like this one some day."

"You can have one!" Charles replied enthusiastically. "Thomas' Uncle Robert has nine more pups that are brothers and sisters of this one." Emily and Sara exchanged excited glances as Charles added; "I would surely love it if you two young ladies each had a pup, because then your pups and mine could grow up as playmates." With a smile, Sara pinched Sly's wrinkled face, giving him a big kiss right on the lips.

"That would be very nice indeed!" Sara replied excitedly. "I do hope our father will allow it! As soon as we get home, I shall ask our father if we can have a pup."

A sad look suddenly came over Emily's face as she remembered asking her father for a dog two years earlier. At that time, her father said to her and Sara, "Now young ladies, a dog is a big responsibility. I am sorry, but I must say no!"

Emily, disappointed, looked at Sara and Charles. "Sad to say, I do not think our father will let us have a pup."

Sara also remembered what her father had said. She looked at the ground, frowning, and said, "Yes, unfortunately, my sister is right."

All of a sudden, Charles' eyes lit up wide with an idea. "Wait a moment!" he replied enthusiastically. "Please allow Thomas and me to walk you young ladies home. That way, your father will be able to see how much you love this pup and how appealing he is, which may influence him to say yes."

"'Twould be most kind of you, Charles." Sara replied looking at Charles smiling at him with her beautiful brown eyes. "Emily and I would certainly appreciate that."

Charles blushed as he replied, "My pleasure, young lady!" On the way over to the Sinclair's house, Sara handed Sly to Emily. She held him in her arms and scratched Sly's tummy. Sly looked at her with pure love in his eyes as he licked her on the face.

Then Emily smiled, and with guilt in her eyes, looked at Thomas and Dare saying, "Once again, I am truly sorry for laughing at you and Dare in the past, along with Todd and the rest of my friends. 'Twas wrong of me."

Thomas lifted his hand, and gave a quick wave. "Fret not, my lady. Both Dare and I forgive you. Right mate?" Dare walked in front of Emily, stopping her with an extended paw, and shaking Emily's hand. Seeing this, Thomas smiled and commented, "Look there, I told you Emily, no hard feelings." Emily smiled, touched by the response of Dare and Thomas.

"I am pleased to hear and see that." Then Emily's smile left her face as she talked about Todd. "Sometimes Todd used to mortify me as well. At times, he can be quite juvenile. 'Tis for that reason I did of late end our romance!"

With a sensitive and caring look, Thomas turned his head towards her and looked in her eyes. As they continued walking, he said, "Only a fool would treat a lovely young lady in such a way! My lady deserves much better than that!"

Touched by Thomas' words, Emily gave him a big beautiful smile while she kept looking in his eyes. "If Todd felt as you do, our romance would not have ended. You and your dog are very special! I would really like to be friends with you both." Thomas had had a crush on Emily most of his life, and hearing her say these words, he felt a little tear come from his eye, and quickly looked away for a second, wiping it off his face. Then Thomas turned and looked in Emily's beautiful blue eyes again, answering her with a smile.

"Certainly, my lady! We both would love to be thy friends. Is that not so Dare?"

"Bark! Bark!"

Thomas interpreted Dare's bark. "That means yes, yes!"

Emily smiled saying, "I am quite pleased to hear that." Thomas thought, *"So am I Emily, so am I."*

Emily saw a cat in a tree looking at her. She pointed the cat out to Thomas asking, "Do thine uncle's dogs get on well with cats?"

"Yes," Thomas answered, "if thou dost introduce them at an early age."

Emily and Sara both sighed with relief as Emily said, "Good, because we recently acquired a kitten."

"My first pet was a cat named Rundy," Thomas said reminiscing. "Rundy and my dog Rascal were great friends. We would always cuddle up together at night when it was cold."

Emily and Sara hearing this, both said, "Ah, how adorable!"

Thomas continued, "One day, I spied a lizard and tried to catch it. However, I could not do so. Rundy was watching my efforts, and when I had finished trying, Rundy caught that lizard, carried it to me in his mouth and dropped it by me feet, all without injuring the lizard."

"'Tis Amazing!" Emily replied, amused. "Now that is a splendid way for a pet to show how much it loves its master." Thomas nodded head, looking away from Emily, and holding back tears as he reminisced about how much he loved his two former pets.

After a few seconds Thomas pulled himself together and replied, "I do agree, my lady. 'Twas comical that afterwards, when Rascal saw how happy Rundy had made me, Rascal did the same thing with a lizard. Before I knew it, both pets were bringing me many kinds of amazing creatures, dropping them off at me feet, while they were still alive, I might add."

"What kinds of creatures?" Emily asked, intrigued.

Thomas chuckled and answered, "Those mad pets brought me live rabbits, live frogs, live opossums and live rats. Rundy sometimes even brought me live birds!" On the way to Emily and Sara's house, Thomas and Emily continued talking and listening to one another, getting to know one another better. They made each other laugh as they exchanged funny little stories.

As soon as Emily and Sara arrived home, they took Sly to their father. Sara held Sly up to him as Emily begged, "Oh, father! Pray, give us leave to have one of this dog's brothers or sisters for our own." Mr. Sinclair looked at Sly and petted him, then looked over at Dare. Mr. Sinclair was put off by Dare's unusual looks, just as like most people were when they saw Dare for the first time. He thought, *"There is no way I am going to have a pup that will eventually even remotely resemble like this freak of nature of a dog here. I will be the laughing stock of my neighborhood!"*

Mr. Sinclair answered his daughters with a disappointed face. "I am sorry. A dog is a big responsibility. A dog needs a lot of attention. I really do not think this family is ready for a dog right now."

Hearing this, Emily and Sara both begged even more. "Oh, dear father! Pray, do let us have a pup." Mr. Sinclair looked again at Dare, taking in a deep breath, and feeling bad because he knew how much his daughters wanted a puppy. He thought, *"Alright, we will get a pup, but it will not be a littermate of this freaky looking pup!"*

He said to his daughters, "Not right now. However, I do promise that in the very near future I will bring home a pup for you."

Emily and Sara, both looking very disappointed, replied, "Alright, father we understand; perhaps in the near future." Just then, they all heard chickens making a lot of noise in the distance. They all looked and saw a group of hungry foxes breaking into Mr. Sinclair's chicken coop. The chickens all took off running for their lives as the foxes chased them.

Mr. Sinclair ran as fast as he could towards the chickens, screaming at the foxes at the top of his lungs. "NOOOO! Leave my chickens alone!" Mr. Sinclair knew that there was no way he could get to the chicken coop in time to save half of his chickens. Thomas looked at Dare, who looked back at Thomas, eagerly waiting for his master to give the command. Thomas smiled, knowing that saving Mr. Sinclair's chickens was child's play for Dare. Thomas looked at his dog and gave a quick nod of his head, which meant, "Thou dost know what to do, me mate." Dare took off running as fast as the wind, making a big cloud of dust in Mr. Sinclair's face as he quickly ran past him. Dare scared off all the foxes, and they ran back into the forest. After this, Dare rounded up all the chickens, and chased them all back safely into their chicken coop, right before Mr. Sinclair's very eyes, and before Mr. Sinclair was even able to reach his chicken coop.

With both hands on his knees and gasping for air, Mr. Sinclair watched Dare as the dog walked over to him. Dare sat in front of Mr. Sinclair, face to face, looking in his eyes. Mr. Sinclair had never seen kinder, more loving eyes in his life. He petted Dare on the head, who in exchange, knocked Mr. Sinclair down to the ground, tickling him as he licked face and neck. This made Mr. Sinclair laugh hysterically, while everyone ran over to them.

Thomas shook his head saying, "Alright Dare; thou hast had thy fun. Now leave Mr. Sinclair alone." Thomas offered Mr. Sinclair a hand up. "I am sorry; me dog still thinks he is a pup. He loves to play with people that he likes, and he really likes you." Mr. Sinclair rose to his feet, brushing the dust off of his pants with his hands.

"Apologies are not needed, son," Mr. Sinclair replied. "Your wonderful dog just saved the lives of all of my chickens. For that, I am very grateful to both you and your dog." Mr. Sinclair looked at Dare, who looked back at him, wiggling his tail. Mr. Sinclair sighed with relief, knowing all of his livestock was intact. He put his hands on Thomas and Charles's shoulders and said, "If your parents consent, I would like to invite you and your dogs over tonight for dinner." Charles put his hand on Thomas' shoulder and looked at Mr. Sinclair with a huge smile on his face.

"We shall go home and ask our parents," Charles said enthusiastically. "But I am certain that it will be fine with them. We shall be more than delighted to join you and your wonderful family tonight for dinner." Charles' innocent smile turned into a lovesick one as his eyes glanced over to Sara, looking her up and down. Mr. Sinclair saw this and dramatically grabbed a big ax while making eye contact with Charles.

"I shall go and prepare another chicken tonight for ye young gentlemen!" Charles gulped and swallowed, seeing Mr. Sinclair waving the ax in his hand as he walked over to the chickens.

"Oh, our thanks, Mr. Sinclair," Charles stuttered with fear. "We will be leaving now to tell our parents that we will be joining you tonight for dinner. We shall return shortly."

Mr. Sinclair, feigning a maniacal look, dramatically grabbed a chicken and put it on a block, replying, "Good! I do look forward to having ye young gentlemen tonight for dinner." As Mr. Sinclair pulled his arm back as if to prepare to chop off the chicken's head, Charles and Thomas exchanged fearful glances, then turned and ran. Seeing the lads run off, Mr. Sinclair laughed, holding himself back momentarily from cutting off the chicken's head.

Emily looked at her father and shook her head. "Why didst thou frighten those lads just now? They might not return for dinner."

With a slight chuckle, Mr. Sinclair answered, "Fear not, Princess. I promise, they will be back! I do know what it is to be their age. I just wanted to intimidate them a little. Now ye two young ladies, go inside. It will not be pretty, seeing what I am about to do to our dinner." Emily and Sara turned and went inside. Mr. Sinclair had a nice chicken picked out for the young gentlemen's dinner. As he raised the ax over his head he said, "If those lads get the wrong idea with my daughters," Mr. Sinclair brought the ax down, powerfully chopping off the chicken's head, "this is what will happen to them."

# CHAPTER XIII
# SO MANY TO CHOOSE FROM

On the lads' way home, Charles put his arm around Thomas, and said, "Thou art most certainly a lucky lad, Thomas. Emily truly likes thee, and she does not like many lads."

With a smile on his face, Thomas asked, "Dost thou truly think so?"

Charles answered, "Foolish boy, I do not just *think* she likes thee; I *know* that she likes thee! And her father really likes thee as well, which is an extremely good thing." Charles frowned as he continued, "I, on the other hand, am still trying to win Mr. Sinclair's approval." Thomas chuckled, thinking about the look that Charles had given Sara in front of her father. "What is so amusing?" Charles asked, annoyed.

Thomas answered, "The way thou dost look at Sara in front of her father, as if you are undressing her with thine eyes."

With a cringe, Charles asked, "Do I really look at Sara that way?"

Thomas rolled his eyes as he answered, "Yes, thou dunce, thou didst do so, and several times. That was the reason Mr. Sinclair was so dramatic with his ax! Just be aware of how thou dost look at his daughter and pay more attention to Mr. Sinclair and thou shouldst be fine." Charles was deep in thought, considering what Thomas had just said to him. He kept quiet, thinking hard as they walked the rest of the way home.

When they arrived at Charles' house, he said to Thomas, "My thanks for the advice. I will see thee and Dare in a little while."

Thomas waved as he walked away, and replied, "Any time mate." Thomas then ran as fast as he could all the way home. He told his parents everything that had happened that day, including the invitation that he and Charles had received to dine at the Sinclair's house that night. Thomas' parents were delighted to hear that Thomas had finally made some friends. However, what Thomas told them about the encounter with Lord Riley was very upsetting to his parents, especially to his father, who knew that Lord Riley was a dog fighter. His father was very troubled to hear that Lord Riley had an interest in his brother's dogs. Thomas' father was very irate at the fact that Lord Riley tried to steal Charles' puppy, and had threatened his life. He told his son to have a good time tonight with Charles at the Sinclair's house, but to be careful and to avoid Lord Riley like the plague. When his son wasn't looking, Thomas' father got down on his knees, petted Dare gently on the head, and whispered in his ear:

"Thou art a very good dog. I am very grateful for thee and thy love for my son. Pray watch over him closely. I have a bad feeling that my son may soon encounter a bad situation. I am trusting thee with my son's life." Hearing this, Dare knocked Thomas' father to the floor, and pinned his shoulders to the ground with his paws. With his nose pressed against Thomas' father's nose, Dare stared ever so intently into his eyes. With eyes like fire, he told him telepathically:

"I know exactly what you have just said to me. No force on this earth is stronger than my love for your son. So do not fret about him. I promise you that no harm will come to your son!" Thomas's father understood. He smiled as he wrapped his arms around Dare, closing his eyes and feeling good knowing his son could not be in any greater care than with this dog. For he knew that Dare would give his own life in a heartbeat to protect his son from any harm. Thomas and Dare waved goodbye to his parents as they left to go to Charles' house. Charles was outside his house, eagerly waiting for them. Charles saw Thomas and Dare a mile away. He ran to meet them with Sly in his arms.

"I am truly excited about tonight! What about you?"

"Certainly!" answered Thomas, thinking of Emily's pretty blue eyes, lovely blonde hair, and beautifully feminine form. When they arrived at the Sinclair's, both Emily and Sara jumped up and down with joy, with smiles a mile wide.

"We have some excellent news." Sara said as she approached Charles. "Soon after ye two left, our father suddenly changed his mind about having a puppy. He told us that we could have a dog from Thomas' uncle tomorrow."

With a huge smile, Emily put both hands on Sly's face, and said "We are going to have a pup like thee tomorrow," giving Sly a big kiss right on the lips.

"That is excellent news," Thomas replied enthusiastically. "I am sure my uncle will be very happy to know that one of his dogs is going to a wonderful family like thine and will receive a lot of love."

Charles nodded his head, looking at Sara with desiring eyes, but remembering what Thomas had told him earlier, Charles quickly turned his head and looked at Mr. Sinclair as he said, "I am very grateful that my pup will be able to play with a brother or sister as he grows up."

Thomas added, "Me, too, and we can also get to know each other better."

As he patted the two lads on the shoulders, Mr. Sinclair replied with a smile on his face and an ironic tone, "Me too! Now let us go eat!" (Both lads gulped, feeling Mr. Sinclair's huge hands on their shoulders.) "Mrs. Sinclair cooked a wonderful dinner tonight for us."

That evening over dinner, Mr. and Mrs. Sinclair could see that there was a strong connection between their daughters and the two boys. In fact, the young people reminded them of themselves when they had first started courting some years ago. That night over dinner, Mr. and Mrs. Sinclair exchanged glances often and smiled at each other, having pleasant reminiscences about when they were younger. By the time dinner was over, both Charles and Thomas had won the approval of Mr. and Mrs. Sinclair.

The next morning, Mr. Sinclair took his daughters, Thomas and Charles on his two-horse carriage to Thomas' Uncle Robert's house to buy a puppy. Thomas told Emily, "Thou shalt not be disappointed," as he stepped out of the carriage.

Robert's dogs, hearing Thomas' voice, leaped off the furniture and ran to the door, barking happily and wagging their tails. Seeing this, Robert knew that his favorite nephew Thomas was the only person who could make his dogs so happy and excited.

Happily, Robert leaped out of his seat, saying as he walked over to the door, "I do believe my favorite nephew is here to visit." Charles had just raised his hand in the air to knock when Robert opened the door with a great big smile on his face. A few of Robert's dogs barged out, running over to Thomas.

Seeing his uncle's dogs charging at him full speed, Thomas waved his hands in the air saying, "Good dogs! Slow down! Stop now!" However, the dogs ignored Thomas' request and leaped in the air, tackling him and knocking him to the ground as they licked his face all over. Thomas lay on the ground, laughing from the tickling. "Alright Sly Ann, Blaze, and Butch, I do miss all of ye as well. Pray, let me greet my uncle first. Then I promise that I will play with ye." Thomas rose to his feet, wiping the dust off his clothes that he had picked up when he had been tackled.

Robert walked over to wipe the dust off of Thomas' that he couldn't reach himself, while saying, "'Tis always nice to have my favorite nephew here for a visit." Robert saw Mr. Sinclair, who was being approached by Sly Ann as she wagged her tail. She sniffed him and started to lick his hand as Mr. Sinclair gently petted her on the head. Robert looked slightly shocked. He and Ted Sinclair had grown up together, and in the past, Ted had made some really unpleasant comments about his dogs. Robert was pleasantly surprised, seeing Sly Ann and Ted getting along so well.

As Ted was scratching Sly Ann's back, he looked up at Robert, saying, "You have quite a nice dog here."

"My thanks for that," Robert replied, even more surprised. "It seems that Sly Ann likes you, Ted. You should feel honored, because she does not like just anybody!" After petting Sly Ann, Ted walked over to Robert with his hand extended.

"I do suppose that dogs just take a liking to me," Ted said as he shook Robert's hand. "Oh, by the way, in the past, when we were young lads, I did say unkind things about your dogs that I do hope you did not take to heart, because 'twas all in jest, you know. If my words were hurtful to you, I do apologize."

Robert wasn't one to hold a grudge. With a dismissive wave of his hand, he shook his head and replied, "Oh no, certainly not." Robert invited Ted and everyone else to come inside his house to sit down and talk. Ted gladly accepted Robert's offer. He walked into Robert's house and looked around, nodding in approval as he saw the paintings and drawings of dogs on the wall. Robert sat down. However, the youngsters did not sit down, nor did they feel much like talking. They were ecstatic about picking out a puppy. Knowing this, Robert smiled and whispered in Thomas' ear, "Take your friends out to the yard. Play tug of war with the dogs for a few minutes, to help calm them down. After thou hast finished playing with the dogs, take the young ladies to the barn and let them pick out their lucky new family member." (Robert whispered this to Thomas because he didn't want Ted to know that he knew that they were there to pick out a puppy. Robert wanted to hear from Ted himself.)

"Many thanks, Uncle Robert," Thomas replied, as he left the room with his friends to go see the dogs. Thomas got a long rope. The youngsters all played tug of war on one end of the rope against Thomas' uncle's dogs on the other end. The four dogs were winning against the youngsters until Dare stepped in to help out his master's team, who then had no problem winning. The four dogs hung onto the rope as Dare dragged them on the ground for a long distance. Dare knew that like himself, his cousins had locking jaws and would not let go of the rope unless they were badly injured. Therefore, Dare let go of the rope for fear that his cousins might get injured because they would not let go.

Meanwhile, Robert spoke to Ted inside the house. "It has been a while. What brings you and your daughters by?" Ted leaned back in his chair. His hands were folded together behind his head, as he remembered some of the things he had said to Robert in the past. Ted felt guilty about things he had said, and wished he could take all of his comments back, but of course he could not.

So Ted humbly told Robert, "My daughters love Charles's pup. I was told that you have more pups, his brothers and sisters. I also did learn from experience that your dogs are excellent herding dogs. That is why I have come here with my daughters. We would like to purchase a pup from you."

Hearing this brought joy to Robert. "Indeed, you have come to the right place." Robert responded enthusiastically. "I do not wish to sound boastful, but I have been told that my dogs are the best working dogs in the world. I would be honored to sell a pup to you and your daughters!" Ted was a bit surprised to hear this, because he knew that Robert didn't just let his dogs go to anybody. Ted knew a few people who had tried to purchase a dog from Robert, but reported that Robert had turned them down. These people said they were denied by some kind of pathetic test. Ted was not aware that he had already passed Robert's test when he and his daughters won Sly Ann's approval. Ted thought that deep down, Robert might still hold a grudge against him for things he had said to Robert in the past. Ted was pleasantly surprised to learn that he was mistaken about this.

Robert soon rose from his chair and walked over to the first picture on the wall. "I would like to tell you a few stories about your future pup's ancestors, if you would care to hear about them."

Ted enthusiastically answered, "Yes! Indeed I would love to hear stories about your dogs!" Hearing this, Robert talked and talked. He talked about Noble, his great ancestor's first dog. Then he walked over to the next picture and talked about Ruffian, his great ancestor's second dog. Ted listened with great interest. Robert then walked over to the third picture and talked about that dog for about an hour, and so on and so on. Finally, after talking for seven hours nonstop about his dog's ancestors, Robert noticed Ted staring at the same spot for a very long time with a slack jaw. Robert could tell that Ted was becoming extremely bored.

"We should see how it goes with your daughters." Robert finally said. "Let us see if they have selected a pup yet." However, Ted did not respond. His mind was in blah, blah land, and he continued to stare at the same spot on the wall. Robert waved his hand in front of Ted's eyes, causing him to come out of his trance.

Ted's head snapped back stunned. "Oh, yes! I hear you! Very interesting story about Clara Bell. Pray, tell me more."

With a slight chuckle, Robert thought, " I have just about driven Ted completely mad. 'Twas over four hours ago that I told the story about Clara Bell." Robert gave Ted a hand out of his chair. "Perhaps I shall tell you that story some other time. Now, let us see how it goes with your daughters." When they walked out in the yard, they immediately saw Emily and Sara rolling around on the ground and laughing while the puppies tickled them by licking their faces and feet. The puppies were wagging their tales while they pulled on the girls' clothes.

"Well young ladies, have ye decided which pup ye want?" asked their father.

"Why yes, good father, we have," Emily answered. "We have decided that we want all of them!"

Their father sighed. "I am sorry, young ladies. You can only have one!" The girls rose to their feet begging.

"Oh, pray father! Let us have them all!"

Once again, their father's response was, "No!"

"Oh please father. We do not wish to take any of them away from their brothers and sisters! Do consider how much happier they all will be, growing up together and playing with each other."

The girls continued to beg, even though their father firmly told them again, "The answer is still no!" Mr. Sinclair turned to Thomas and Charles as he continued, "Besides, I am sure thy young gentlemen friends will come to our home often with their dogs for your pup to play with. Right lads?"

Charles responded, nodding his head with a mischievous smile. "Oh-yes! Most definitely!"

Sara began to act like she was crying. "But father."

Her father quickly interrupted her, "Alright young ladies, we shall now go home with no pup!"

Sara quickly changed her tone. "One pup will be fine, father, our thanks."

"I thought so!" her father replied, smirking. "Have my daughters now made their decision about which pup they want?" As the girls looked back at the litter, the puppies were all sitting and wagging their tails, staring at the girls with cute puppy dog eyes as if to say, "Please, choose me! I will be a good dog. I will always love you."

The girls looked back at their father answering, "Ah- we shall need a little more time to decide."

Mr. Sinclair shook his head gasping, "Oh, no! 'Tis going to be a long day." After about an hour, the girls decided on a female puppy. Emily named her Liena, because the puppy moved like a lion cub. Her father chuckled at this name his daughter made up as he pulled out his money. "Robert, how much do I owe you for Liena?"

Robert answered, "You pay me whatever you want. I never breed dogs for money, just for companions and helpers on my farm." Mr. Sinclair nodded his head, impressed.

"I appreciate that; however, I do insist on paying you seven-shillings for my daughter's pup!" This was about five times the amount of money that most people normally paid for a dog. Mr. Sinclair felt guilty about all the times he had made fun of Robert's dogs when they were kids, which was why he offered so much money for Liena. This was Ted's way of clearing his conscience for all the times he hurt Robert's feelings when they were growing up together. Robert gladly accepted Ted's offer. He gave the Sinclair's some food for Liena and gave the dog a kiss on the head as he always did whenever he said goodbye to one of his dogs. Robert was all choked up inside, for he was sad to see Liena go, but also because once again Robert knew one of his pups was going to a good home.

As they left, Robert shouted towards Mr. Sinclair's carriage, "Do not be strangers! Come by anytime," and waved goodbye.

Emily shouted back, "Many thanks, we will!" then she looked directly across her seat at Thomas, asking with a flirtatious look, "Will we not?"

Thomas answered with a slight blush, "Yes, my lady!" and whispered softly with his breath, "I will go anywhere with thee."

Immediately after Robert walked in his house with Blaze and closed his door Dare smelled a familiar scent that was extremely displeasing. His back hairs all rose up as he moved his flared nostrils side to side smelling. When Dare locked unto the vicinity of the scent, he leaped out of the carriage, running towards the river, violently barking in attack mode. Mr. Sinclair halted his horses and they all followed Dare on foot. "What is wrong, mate?" Thomas asked, catching his breath as he finally caught up to his dog. His friends soon also caught up, and looked all around as Dare continued to bark violently as he looked up and down the river.

"I do not see anything out here," Charles commented. "He probably smelled an animal and chased it into the river. It is probably long gone by now and on the other side."

However, Thomas wasn't so sure. He looked around the area with a skeptical expression on his face as Dare kept barking. Eventually, Thomas gave up. He tried to calm Dare down by patting him on the head while saying, "Come Dare, 'tis alright. Whatever it was is probably gone." Dare reluctantly turned around with his master and friends and followed them back to Mr. Sinclair's carriage. As soon as they left the area, Lord Riley's head popped out of the water and he gasped for air. He was staking out Thomas' uncle's place, and planning to steal Blaze to use as a stud dog, in hopes of producing more dogs just like Terror.

# CHAPTER XIV
# THE BIG ONE

On their way home, Thomas said, "I say we should all go fishing tomorrow. It looks like it may rain, which is the best time to go."

Charles quickly responded, "Thou canst be certain I will go. How about ye two, young ladies?"

"May we go?" Sara asked her father.

"There is no way that I would allow it!" Her father answered firmly as he looked intensely at Thomas and Charles. "'Tis unsafe if it rains, and I do not wish for my daughters to take sick. I do not recommend that ye two lads go tomorrow either. However, I am not your father, so I shall not tell ye lads what to do. However, if ye two ever wish to see my daughters again, ye will come to your senses and not go fishing tomorrow, either, if it rains."

Charles and Thomas looked shocked to hear this from Mr. Sinclair. Charles quickly responded out of fear. "I do agree with you, Mr. Sinclair. 'Twould be rather foolish to fish in the rain. I do not know what we were thinking. Pray forgive us for Thomas' foolish thoughts."

"Huh," Thomas replied as he cringed, surprised at being the main object of blame.

At the same time, Sara raised her voice at her father, saying "Good father, you do not have the right to threaten the young gentlemen."

"Thou art right, Sara," her father responded, chuckling before addressing Thomas and Charles again. "I am only jesting with ye lads. Ye can still visit my daughters, whether or not ye go fishing in the rain." Charles felt like a brown nose for buttering up Sara's father. However, the girls knew that their father's answer was not negotiable.

Therefore, Emily told Thomas and Charles, "Our thanks for your kind offer. We would love to go fishing with ye, along with our dogs, but we cannot. I promise that we will go some other time, but not in the rain."

Hearing this, Emily's father smiled, proud of his daughters. "I do wish ye good luck fishing tomorrow," Mr. Sinclair told Thomas and Charles as he dropped them off near Charles' home. "If the two of ye decide to go, I hope that ye catch many fish."

"Our thanks, Mr. Sinclair," Charles answered as he and Thomas waved and said their goodbyes.

As the Sinclairs rode home, Thomas patted Charles on the shoulder. "Well mate, looks like 'twill just be us and our dogs fishing tomorrow."

Charles looked up that moment and saw some thick clouds in the distance,"Yes! It does appear that it will be only us two." Charles said this reluctantly, swallowing hard, looking perturbed, and then added, "It certainly does look like it might rain very hard tomorrow. Art thou certain that thou dost still want to go fishing, even without the damsels?"

"Of course I am certain!" Thomas answered with conviction. "Right before a storm is the best time to go fishing."

"All right, then, mate," Charles replied. "Sly and I shall see thee first thing in the morning."

" Excellent," Thomas responded, looking slightly upset, knowing that Charles was having second thoughts. "'Tis my custom to set out just before the sun rises."

Hearing this, Charles whistled unenthusiastically as he walked up to his front door. "Good grief, 'tis very early. However, Sly and I shall be ready," Charles said as he and Sly walked into their house.

The next morning, Thomas and Dare woke up very early. The clouds were thick and dark, looking like they were going to start dropping rain like buckets at any minute. It was already sprinkling. Thomas and Dare walked over to Charles' house. When they arrived, Charles was still asleep. Thomas knocked on the door, waking up Charles, along with his mother, who in turn woke up her husband, who answered the door.

"What dost thou want?" asked Charles' father, irritated at being awakened.

Just then, Charles came to the door yawning, and said, "Tis alright father. I did promise my friend Thomas that I would go fishing with him today."

Charles' father looked outside. He heard the rumble of thunder and saw thick rain clouds, "Not today! Thou shalt not go fishing today, son! It looks like a heavy rain is about to come down." Charles' father paused, sighing, "I tell thee, think not to fish today!"

Charles looked at Thomas and saw a very disappointed look on his face. Feeling guilty, Charles pleaded, "Oh father, pray do let me go. Yesterday I gave Thomas my word that this morning I would go fishing with him."

Charles' father shook his head no. He was both tired and angry. "Well son, thou shouldst not have promised that, knowing that there was a good chance of a big storm today."

"No, father," Charles answered with his head hung low.

Charles' father continued scolding, "Get thy carbuncled bottom to thy bed chambers this instant, young whelp! And not another word!"

Charles knew that his father was very angry and also knew that nothing that he could say would make his father change his mind. Feeling extremely guilty, Charles told Thomas, "Sorry mate, but I can not go fishing with thee today"

Thomas was disappointed, but responded, "I understand."

Charles quickly glanced at his father, when he wasn't looking, and turned around and went back to bed.

Charles' father yawned, and put his hand on Thomas' shoulder. Sensing perhaps a touch of hostility towards his son, he said, "Pray, do not be angry at my son. He is a good lad and a person of his word. I am sorry, but I cannot allow him to go. I do hope you understand that I care much for him. Perhaps thou shouldst reconsider fishing today. It may not be safe out there!"

Thomas thanked Charles' father for his advice, and apologized for waking his family up, but he did not heed his warning. In fact, as he and Dare continued towards their favorite fishing spot, Thomas shook his head and laughed as he thought about Charles' father.

Thomas soon ended up at a field at Lord Riley's farm. His father knew that going through that field was a short cut to their favorite fishing spot, and had strictly forbidden Thomas to ever go through that field. Lurking in the field at times was a humungous bull named Bulldread. Six times he had survived fighting in the pit, killing several bulldogs. Thomas, with no Bulldread in sight and pressed for time, ignored his father's command for the first time in his life. Even Dare knew that they were not supposed to cross through Lord Riley's field, and he barked as Thomas crawled underneath the fence. "Quiet!" Thomas ordered as he continued looking around, "Bulldread is nowhere in sight. Come now, live up to your name." Dare obeyed his master as always, this time reluctantly. Quickly, they ran across Lord Riley's field and safely reached the other side. They soon ended up at their favorite fishing spot, where Thomas threw out his line and instantly caught a big trout.

"Most excellent, Dare," Thomas said with excitement. "It seems this is to be our lucky day." Shortly after that, Thomas caught five more fish. Thomas sat on a log with Dare by his side, watching over him as always. He put his arm around Dare as the two stared at a beautiful rainbow, seen at a far distance as the sun rose. Thomas said," Dare, I want thee to know that thou art me best mate, the best in the whole world. I cannot always count on people to help me, or to accept me for myself. However, I can always count on thee to do that and to love me no matter what. I want thee to know, Dare, I shall always love thee no matter what, as well."

Dare turned away from the beautiful rainbow and sunrise and looked at his master, licking his face as if to say, "I understand what you hast just said to me. I do feel the same way, too, and am the world's luckiest dog to have a master like you."

A short while later, the distant rainbow was replaced by thick, dark storm clouds, and the whole sky now became cloudy and dark. It began to rain hard, as the sky lit up with lightning, and rumbled with loud thunder.

Thomas turned to Dare, saying "Well mate, 'tis time for us to leave." Just after Thomas said this and was about to bring in his line, he got a strong bite, much stronger than any bite he had ever gotten before. The sky lit up with lightning and rumbled even more at that moment. "Hold on Dare! I think we have one more fish to bring in," Thomas said ecstatically. He jumped to his feet and struggled for about an hour to bring in the fish, without even seeing it. When Thomas eventually saw the fish, his eyes widened and his mouth opened in disbelief. This was the biggest fish he had ever seen in his life. Meanwhile, the sky flashed with lightning and rumbled with thunder. As the fish got closer to shore, it fought even harder, taking Thomas' line back out again. But the big fish was starting to get tired, as was Thomas. However, Thomas' adrenaline kept him going and gave him extra strength. A few minutes later, he saw the fish again. Thomas screamed with excitement! "Look thou, Dare, at that huge fish! We are about to catch it!"

Then he made a big mistake. The fish was almost on shore. Overwhelmed with excitement, Thomas pulled too hard on his line, causing the huge fish to come out of the water and the hook to come out of his mouth, merely inches away from shore. Thomas fell backwards and sat down hard, feeling like a dagger pierced threw his heart. With wide eyes, he watched helplessly as the monstrous fish flopped back into the water, about to swim away.

Dare, knowing the importance of this fish to his master, instantly reacted. He plunged face first into the water, and biting the fish on the bottom lip with his left two fangs, he lifted his head up out of the water, and pulled the fish out also. With his powerful neck muscles, Dare twisted his neck, throwing the monstrous fish on his master's stomach. This felt like a wonderful punch in the stomach, causing the wind to be knocked out of Thomas for a second. He gasped for air as he wrapped his arms around the monstrous fish, which was flapping in his arms, almost as big as he was. Laughing hysterically, he screamed. "Halleluiah! We did it, Dare, we did it! We caught the biggest fish ever!" Dare jumped out of the water, running over to his master and licked his face as he wagged his tail. For whenever his master was happy, Dare was happy. Thomas was still on the ground, laughing and holding the fish, with the rain coming down on him like buckets of water. Thomas eventually rose to his feet, never losing his smile. Overwhelmed with joy, he grabbed Dare's wrinkled cheeks as he gave him a big kiss right on the lips. "Many thanks, me best mate." Then, tasting a drop of saliva, he grimaced and spit. Then he said, "I could not have caught this fish without thee. Let us now bring it home and astound everyone!" This was by far the best fishing day Thomas had ever had. The weight of all the fish was impossible for him to carry, so he left some of the fish on the ground and started to walk home.

As he started to leave, Dare barked, looking at the fish on the ground. "What is wrong, Dare?" Thomas asked, "Wouldst thou like to carry some of the fish home?"

Dare barked as if to answer, "Why yes, I would. 'Tis not right that any good fish go to waste." So, Thomas put the huge fish on Dare's back and tied some line around it. Dare carried the fish with no problem.

Thomas looked at Dare with his big smile remaining, "Thou art a special dog! We shall now have plenty of fish to give to my Uncle Robert, and to some other people who are close to us." Thomas picked up the rest of the fish and headed towards home.

Meanwhile, Charles felt very guilty because he had not gone fishing with Thomas and Dare. He wanted to make sure that their friendship was intact, so he put on his clothes for the rain and told his parents that he was just going over to Thomas' house to see how he had done fishing.

Charles' father, squinting, reluctantly agreed. "Very well, my son, but be careful and do not be long."

"I shall, good father," Charles replied as he left his house to walk towards Thomas's home.

When Charles arrived, Thomas' mother answered the door. She told Charles, "My son and Dare are still out fishing."

"Astounding," Charles replied concerned, "They certainly have been gone a long time."

Thomas' mother nodded her head. "Yes, indeed they have. They should be home any time now."

Thomas' father came to the door. "Greetings, Charles. Thou art welcome to come inside and wait for Thomas, if thou dost so desire."

"Many thanks, but no, Mr. Gentry," Charles answered. "I do think I shall go to meet your son on his way home and help him carry his things." Charles walked away a little stunned that Thomas' parents did not seem very concerned about him. Thomas's parents, however, knew that their son was in good hands with Dare. Charles headed towards Thomas' favorite fishing spot to see how he was doing, or to meet him on his way home.

At this moment, Thomas and Dare reached Lord Riley's field. Thomas looked all around the field for any bulls, but he couldn't see very well because it was very dark due to the rain and thick clouds. So, he thought they would play it safe and take the long way home by walking around Lord Riley's field. Just as Thomas started to walk with Dare, lightning suddenly lit up the sky again, giving Thomas a good clear look at Lord Riley's field. Since there were no bulls in sight, Thomas thought it would be safe for them to cross the field, so he turned around, came back and crawled underneath Lord Riley's fence. "Come on Dare, tis safe for us to cross."

However, Dare was hesitant, sensing that something was wrong. Reluctantly, he crawled underneath the fence, and then looked around the field ever so cautiously while walking with his master. When they were nearly half way across the field, lightning struck, lighting up the field again. This time, Lord Riley happened to be looking over his field while he was on his way to the barn to feed his livestock. Lord Riley spotted Thomas and Dare, who saw Lord Riley looking at them with furious eyes. Thomas knew he had made a big mistake. Panicking, he started to run across the field.

Dare ran along side of his master, barking at him as if to say, "Slow down!

'Tis dark, muddy, and slippery, and thou art carrying heavy things. 'Tis not safe to be running right now!" Thomas, however, did not heed his dog's warning to slow down, and stepped in a large gofer hole, which caused him to trip and fall in the mud. He quickly tried to get up, but couldn't because his ankle was severely sprained. Falling back in the mud, he pulled his leg close to his chest. Holding his ankle, he screamed out in agony, while lightning flashed and thunder rumbled.

# CHAPTER XV
# LEAVE MY CARROT ALONE

Seeing Thomas lying helpless in the mud, Lord Riley thought, *"It serves him right! I do not like anyone to use my property as a short cut. I have seen this bastard and his dog do this earlier. Therefore, I shall make bloody sure they never set foot on my property again!"* With his hand to his chin and narrowing his beady eyes, he contemplated his options. *"Hmm, what should I do? My dog Terror seems to have no problem killing bulls, with the help of a few other strong dogs. I have often wondered how Terror would do if I put him in a pit by himself to fight a bull, but have feared that Terror would get killed. This would be a real tragedy to me, especially because I do not yet have any really powerful offspring from him yet. However, if I could see his brother fight alone against a huge bull such as Bulldread, I would have a good idea of how Terror would do."* Lord Riley's fiendish thoughts began to emerge. *"Now to get a bull to fight Terror's brother, I shall walk over to the barn, where lives one of the biggest, meanest bulls on the planet, and open the barn door."* Lord Riley did so, letting Bulldread out into his field. Next, Lord Riley showed Bulldread his favorite food, a big juicy carrot, held the carrot up to Bulldread's nose and teased him with it. "See this big juicy carrot? I know thou dost want it."

Bulldread smelled the carrot. Grunting, he opened up his mouth, trying to chomp on the carrot. Lord Riley, however, pulled the carrot away just as Bulldread was about to chomp on it. Lord Riley then did a really mean trick to infuriate Bulldread. He quickly switched the carrot to his left hand, while holding a rock in his right hand. Bulldread still thought Lord Riley was holding the carrot in his right hand. Next, Lord Riley threw the rock at Thomas and Dare, almost hitting them.

Bulldread thought that Lord Riley had thrown the carrot instead of the rock.

With his devilish smile, Lord Riley looked at Bulldread saying, "Well, go get it!" Bulldread ran towards Thomas and Dare.

Aware of Bulldread, Dare quickly and powerfully shook his body, causing the string tied around his back to snap. The giant fish he was carrying flopped to the ground, as Dare began to bark louder then he ever had in his whole life. He was fully prepared to fight to the death as he stood in front of his beloved master, who lay helpless in the mud. Hearing Dare's loud and furious barks, Bulldread stopped. At first, he did not think Dare was a dog because the barks he heard sounded more like a lion roaring than a dog barking. Also, the way Dare moved, so agile and loose was more like a big cat than a dog. Bulldread saw Dare's gigantic fangs that were sticking out of his mouth, looking like they could crush the thickest of bones with ease. Bulldread had never seen such fangs before in any dog. Bulldread was very hungry and wanted the carrot, which he thought was near Thomas and Dare, but was very intimidated by Dare. Bulldread knew full well, by the gleaming look of fire in the dog's eyes, that if he did engage in a fight, it would be a fight to the death. Therefore, Bulldread circled around Thomas and Dare, looking for any signs of weakness that his adversaries might have. Dare circled as Bulldread circled. He stood in front of his master. Dare had no regard for his own life, but only for the life of his master.

After a few seconds of the circling, Thomas ordered Dare to leave, yelling, "Go get help, Dare! There is no use in both of us dying! I now command thee to leave at once and get help!"

For the first time in his life, Dare did not obey his master's command. Thomas continued to command Dare to leave, but to no avail. Thomas soon forced himself to his feet. In great agony, he limped over to Dare and began slapping him in the face. His tears fell to the ground like the rain that was coming down as he screamed, "Thou must listen to me, dumb dog! I do not love thee, nor have I ever loved thee. So go! Leave now! And do not look back!" These words didn't mean anything to Dare, for he knew his master's heart, and knew without a shadow of a doubt that his master loved him. However, Dare realized that there was no way he would have any chance of saving his master's life if his master kept slapping him in the face and yelling at him. Dare knew Bulldread was more likely to attack them both if his master kept this up. Also, Dare would not be able to see Bulldread charge at them too well either. Dare wanted to get his master out of there unharmed more than anything in the world. But at this point, the best thing Dare could do for his master was to obey him, just like always, so Dare calmly and slowly walked away, with his head down and his tail between his legs.

Dare looked at his master with a very hurt look in his eyes, which were crying out, "Pray, do not send me away right now master. Thou dost need me by thy side right now more than thou ever hast in thine entire life." However, Thomas continued to let his dog walk away, thinking that this huge bull was going to attack. Thomas assumed that he was about to die and so there was no point in his dog dying also. Half a minute later lightning lit up the sky again. This time, Dare was nowhere in sight. Thomas fell back into the mud, grabbing his badly sprained ankle as he cried out in agony. He was relieved that his dog was away from danger, but at the same time he felt great sorrow, for he had not expected his dog to forsake him so quickly, leaving him there to die alone.

Lord Riley watched all this with great intensity, wanting very much to see the outcome of the fight to the death between Bulldread and Terror's brother. However, after seeing Dare turn and walk away, Lord Riley did not think that this was going to happen. He became furious and clinched his fists in rage, yelling in disbelief at Dare, "Thou cowardly disgrace of a creature! Come back and fight! Do not tell me thou art going to let thy master get killed without at least trying to save his life! If thou dost this, thou shalt be the biggest disgrace in animal history! So return and fight, thou bloody son of a bitch."

Hearing Lord Riley, Thomas began to cry and plead for his help, "Pray show mercy, my Lord! I am sorry for trying to cross through your field! It shall never happen again! For God's sake, do not let your bull kill me!"

Lord Riley just looked Thomas in the eye, giving an evil grin as if to say, "Save your breath, stupid lad. 'Twould be better to have thought about that before ever setting foot on my property! 'Twill be a pleasure to watch thee die!" As the lightning flashed again, Thomas got a really good look deep into Lord Riley's eyes and through the gateway of his soul, saw that Lord Riley's spirit was filled with utter evil. Lord Riley picked up a stick as he turned his back on Thomas and began carving the stick with his knife. Thomas knew that Lord Riley was not going to lift a finger to save his life. So, rather than begging for Lord Riley's help, which would accomplish nothing, Thomas raised his head, folded his hands, and prayed for God's help. Lord Riley watched Thomas praying out of the corner of his eye. He shook his head thinking what a stupid lad. He would be much better off trying to crawl for his life, rather than wasting valuable time and energy praying to a God that does not exist.

Bulldread, angry and hungry, continued to circle Thomas, looking and sniffing for the carrot that he believed Lord Riley had thrown out there. After hard searching and sniffing, Bulldread stopped moving and looked at Thomas. With an angry look on his face, Bulldread came to one conclusion. Thomas had eaten the carrot. Bulldread became enraged at Thomas. He circled Thomas a few more times. Now, Bulldread was no longer intimidated about attacking Thomas, because Dare was nowhere to be seen. Bulldread saw no sign of a dangerous fight. Suddenly, he stopped circling, put his head low to the ground, and with his right hoof, kicked mud back. Bulldread was now ready to attack.

Just at this moment, Charles arrived as lightning lit up the sky again. He saw Thomas lying helplessly in the mud and Bulldread about to charge.

Seeing Charles, Lord Riley opened the barn door to Bulldread's pen, and went inside, closing the door before he was seen by Charles. Lord Riley kept hidden and looked out through a little peephole, because he did not want Charles to see him watching his bull kill Thomas, for fear that Charles might tell the townspeople that he was a murderer. So Lord Riley said to himself as he continued to hide, *"When Bulldread kills this bloody little bastard, I shall act ignorant, as if I did not know it happened, and had nothing to do with it."*

Charles quickly crawled beneath Lord Riley's fence and picked up a rock to throw at Bulldread. Charles was trying to get Bulldread's attention and induce the animal to approach himself instead, with the hope that he would be able to get his friend out of there safely. Charles, however, was a little too late. Before he had time to get Bulldread's attention, Bulldread started his charge at Thomas.

Thomas saw Bulldread charging at him and thought, *"My life is about to end."* Thomas looked up in the sky yelling, "My God, save me!"

At that very moment, lightning lit up the sky more than ever. For the next few seconds, everything for miles around was clearly visible. Bulldread was just a couple of seconds away from ending Thomas' life by spearing the boy with his horns. Charles closed his eyes and began to cover them with his hands, when suddenly he saw what he thought was an angelic creature, because it moved faster than the wind and came out from nowhere. This creature sped towards Bulldread and Thomas, who was on his back with his eyes wide open, with the rain falling in them as he looked up at the sky. However, for a fraction of a second, the rain didn't fall in his eyes. The creature that Charles saw jumped directly over the top of Thomas' head, sheltering his' eyes momentarily from the rain with his body. What Charles thought was an angelic creature was in reality Thomas' faithful dog Dare. Thomas glimpsed at his dog's stomach, his dog's legs and arms fully extended about nine feet above his head. Dare looked like nothing of this earth, for he moved with lightning speed as he came to his masters' rescue. Dare was extremely angry. There was no force on this earth that was stronger than the love he had for his beloved master. Dare had never abandoned his master, nor did he have any intentions of doing so. He had been hiding behind a tree, knowing that Bulldread was less likely to attack if Thomas kept calm. Unfortunately, this didn't work. Dare also knew if he had to fight Bulldread, he would be able to attack more effectively without his master yelling, slapping and distracting him. Dare was now in full force attack mode and focused on Bulldread one hundred percent. As Dare jumped over his master, his mouth was wide open and his razor sharp fangs were fully exposed. He looked and moved like a big cat, rather than a dog. Bulldread saw this and was disturbed and surprised.

He tried to stop, but couldn't. Before Dare hit the ground, his jaws collided with Bulldread's nose, making a very loud sound that could have been easily mistaken for the sound of the loud thunder above them. As soon as the animals collided, blood spurted out of Bulldread's nose, and a lot of it splattered onto Thomas' face. He was just a few feet away. Dare locked his jaws onto Bulldread's nose and held on in mid air. Bulldread's feet skidded, stopping just an inch away from Thomas, who would have been crushed had Bulldread stepped on him. Bulldread violently shook his head back and forth directly over Thomas. Desperately, Bulldread tried to shake off this crazy, intense dog, as more blood spewed out of his nose and dripped into Thomas' face and eyes. Thomas just lay on the ground in shock, staring up as he watched his dog being swung back and forth like a rag doll. As Bulldread's huge horns barely missed him he thought, *"This is not happening; I am in a bad dream and am about to wake up any second now."* However, this nightmare was a reality, and Thomas could not escape by waking up.

Watching all this in awe, Charles dropped his rock along with his jaw! Lord Riley also dropped his knife as he, too, looked on awestruck. Bulldread soon moved away from Thomas, and kept shaking his head back and forth, trying to get Dare off of his nose. Dare kept his jaws locked on, fighting for his master's life. Then Dare was thrown twelve feet into the air, directly over the top of Bulldread, as Bulldread's nose came off, along with a big piece of nose cartilage and skin. Dare landed directly on top of Bulldread, near the bull's neck, and was able to bite Bulldread's jugular vain. Bulldread continued to shake, but less than he had before, because he was weakening from the loss of blood gushing out of his nose. Bulldread eventually fell to the ground. With every ounce of strength he had, Dare pulled his head up, ripping a chunk of Bulldread's neck out, along with a piece of jugular vain. After this, Dare collapsed on the ground. In great pain, Bulldread rose to his feet again, as he made a painful moaning sound. Then Bulldread charged at Thomas, who still lay helpless in the mud. When Bulldread came just inches away from Thomas, he suddenly collapsed on the ground again, and this time did not get up, for Bulldread died when he hit the ground, creating a pool of blood, which even the thick rain wasn't able to wash away.

# CHAPTER XVI
# CRACKING BONES!

Thomas saw Dare lying on the ground, trying desperately to move. Thomas knew that his beloved dog was badly injured and needed help right away. Quickly, he grabbed one of Bulldread's horns, using it to help him rise to his feet. Upon taking two steps towards Dare, though, he slipped because of the water mixed with Bulldread's blood and started falling face downwards again. At this moment Charles approached, sprinting over. With lightning reflexes, he caught his friend, preventing him from splashing in the bloody mud.

"Art thou badly injured, mate?" Charles asked concerned, especially seeing his friend drenched with blood from head to toe.

"No!" Thomas convincingly answered. "Dare is, though! He must be tended to at once!" Charles helped his literally bloody friend over to Dare. Thomas dropped to his knees, gently wrapping his arms around his best friend crying out loud. "I love thee, Dare! Hear me! Thou must pull through! Do not die! Keep fighting!"

While lying on the ground in great pain, Dare slowly turned his eyes upward looking at his master. However, no matter how great his pain was, a happy look sparkled in his eyes, for he knew he had just saved his master's life. Thomas saw the love and pain in his dog's eyes and started to panic. Desperately, Thomas tried to lift Dare up, but couldn't even lift himself up off the ground. After a few failed attempts, he wrapped his arms back around Dare crying like a baby, saying over and over, "Do not die, Dare! Do not die!" Charles, on the other hand, did not panic. Thinking fast and intelligently, he pulled out his knife, took off his shirt, and cut it into a few big pieces. Next, he wrapped the pieces around Dare's worst cuts to help stop the bleeding. Charles looked all around for something he could use to move Dare, but found nothing. Suddenly, lightening lit up the sky again, enabling him to see a nice big wheel barrow, which could be used to move Dare. Quickly, Charles ran over to take it. As his hand reached out to grab one of the wheelbarrow handles, the sky lit up again. This time a cold chill ran down his spine, for standing directly in front of him, holding the other handle of the wheelbarrow, was Lord Riley.

"What art thou doing on my property?" he asked harshly "Art thou trying to steal my wheelbarrow?" "No, my Lord," Charles answered, trembling as he looked up and saw the rage in the evil Lord's eyes. He attempted reasoning, "Pray forgive me for the intrusion, my Lord. I have no intentions of stealing your wheelbarrow. I only wish to borrow it! Me mate and his dog are badly injured and need tending to at once!"

Lord Riley replied without compassion, "Well now, I do warrant that they should not have been trespassing on my land!"

"Pray show mercy, my lord!" Charles pleaded, taking out three shillings from his pocket. "This is yours for your kindness, in letting us borrow your wheel barrow," he said this handing Lord Riley the shillings. "This is more than enough to buy your wheelbarrow, but I am only borrowing it. However, if milord feels this is not enough, I will gladly pay much more when I return your wheel barrow."

With a demonic grin, Lord Riley looked at the money in his hand and said, "My answer is no! This money is mine regardless"

At that point, Charles knew that the only way to get the wheelbarrow was to scare Lord Riley. So he backed up, threatening in an angry tone, "If you do not give me leave to borrow your wheelbarrow, me mate and his dog may die here. If this happens, I swear by all that is holy that I shall tell the whole town that you killed them!"

Seeing Thomas drenched with blood, Lord Riley assumed that Bulldread had pierced him with his horn and that the young lad and his dog were both soon to die. Lord Riley knew that if Charles made good on his threat, it would mean an awful lot of trouble for himself. Without compassion, he looked over at Thomas, who was still crying as he held his dog in his arms. This sight pleased the wicked Lord Riley. As the lightning lit up the sky again, Lord Riley saw the gigantic fish that Thomas had caught. This was by far the biggest fish he had ever seen. Whistling, with eyes wide, he backed away from the wheelbarrow saying, "Alright! However, I have one condition."

"Name it, milord," Charles replied.

"Thou must leave that big fish that they caught here with me and give me thy word that no one will ever hear of any of this!"

Charles knew that the fish Thomas had caught wasn't even on his mind right now. He nodded his head responding, "So be it, milord. I give you me word!" Then Charles picked up a piece of wood, and put it into the wheelbarrow.

Not wasting any precious time, Charles quickly ran over to his injured friends. He helped Thomas up and gave him the stick he had found for a crutch as he told him. "Thou must pull thyself together now, mate. Thy dog shall be all right!" Thomas stood there, taking in a few deep breaths and calming down, while Charles gently and calmly petted Dare, preparing him to be lifted. Lord Riley was afraid that if word got out that a young lad and his dog had been killed by Bulldread on his estate, his foes in the town who opposed bull baiting would have ammunition to use against him, especially if he did nothing to help or did not even offer assistance. Therefore, with an uncompassionate face, Lord Riley made an insincere effort to help. However, as Lord Riley extended his hands to help Charles put Dare into the wheelbarrow, Dare moved his body, squirming towards Lord Riley and attempted to bite his hands off.

Lord Riley quickly pulled his hands away. "Well excuse the bloody hell out of me! I am merely trying to help!"

As Dare barked, Charles and Thomas both yelled at Lord Riley, "We do not need your bloody help. Leave us at once!"

Lord Riley, acting as if his intentions were pure replied, "So be it. If ye do not wish to have my help, my help ye shall not receive! Oh, by the way Charles, seeing that I am such a gentleman and a generous Lord, there will be no charge for that wheelbarrow, not even one penny." Lord Riley tried to hand the money back to Charles, and as he did so, Dare again tried to lunge at Lord Riley.

Thomas and Charles screamed again at Lord Riley, "Leave us!"

"Fine" Lord Riley responded with an attitude, "'Tis thy loss!" He walked over to the gate of his fence, "At least let me open this for thee." He said opening it, "I shall leave thy three shillings on the fence. Thou mayest take it as thou dost leave." Charles, with all of his strength, gently lifted Dare into the wheelbarrow. The money was completely ignored.

Lord Riley picked up the huge fish with a greedy, sinister smile and slowly walked away whispering, "Foolish bastards. I hope your bloody flesh rots!"

Hearing this, Dare turned, with fangs exposed, looking at the wicked Lord Riley. Knowing that fish meant a lot to his master, Dare growled and barked at Lord Riley and tried to get up to retrieve the fish. Seeing this, Thomas commanded Dare to stay still. Thomas didn't even look at the fish, nor did he think about it. The well being of his dog was the only thing on his mind. He limped along, leaning on the stick that Charles had given him, while Charles pushed Dare over to Thomas' house in the wheelbarrow. When they arrived, Charles ran to the door and told Mr. Gentry a little of what had happened, while Thomas stayed with Dare.

Mr. Gentry quickly grabbed his coat, telling his wife that he was going to his brother's house and would be gone for a while. He ran out to his son to make sure he was all right. After checking on his son, Mr. Gentry wrapped a warm blanket around Dare and gently picked him up, moving him in his horse's carriage, then yelled to his four horses, "Hi, Yah." as he snapped the reins. They quickly rode off towards Robert's house, and on the way, quickly dropped Charles off at his home. Then he urged his horses to run like the wind to his brother's home. When they arrived, Robert was on the porch, eagerly waiting for them. His dogs knew the sound of Thomas' father Justin's four-horse carriage and could hear them coming fast from a half a mile away, even in this storm. It was out of the ordinary for Justin to ride so fast, especially in stormy weather. Roberts's dogs barked loud notifying their master that something was not right. As Justin's carriage pulled up, Robert ran out to meet it in the rain. He noticed Dare was cross eyed in the left eye and badly injured.

Robert took a deep breath and gave a quick whistle, "Well, let us not waste any time. Bring him inside at once. Let us see what we can do for him. I have mended the injuries of many dogs that were hurt while they herded my cattle. Do not fret. I shall do me best to mend him." Deep down inside though he silently prayed as he looked in Dares' eyes, "Lord God, this poor dog is very badly injured. Without Your help, my nephew's dog will surely die." Thomas' father gently moved Dare inside, putting him on a table so they could get a better look at him. Robert's dogs gathered around Dare, licking his wounds. Robert patted his dogs on the head. "All right, Sly Ann, Star and Blaze. I know ye all mean well, but please move away from Dare for the moment. I need to look at him right now." The dogs instantly moved away, for they knew their big friend was badly injured and felt sorry for him. Robert unwrapped the pieces of shirt that Charles had wrapped around Dare's wounds. He complimented the wrapping as he grabbed his alcohol. Softly he spoke to Dare, "This may hurt a little, mate." Dare showed no signs of pain while his wounds were being wiped with the alcohol. Next, Robert took out a needle and some thread. Gently he patted Dare again. "This is truly going to hurt. It is of the utmost importance though for thee to remain still." Robert instructed his nephew, "Keep thine arms around Dare and tell him calmly and repeatedly to hold still while I sew up his wounds." Thomas did so, and Dare flinched a little from the pain, but behaved exceptionally well overall. Robert finished stitching Dare up with no problems. Robert felt Dare's bones. They were badly out of alignment, and there were sprains as well. Robert put Thomas' hands on Dare's back, near the middle, and asked Thomas, "Feel how this one part is not in place with the other part, and how there is a little S shape to his back?"

Thomas answered, "Yes uncle, I do feel it and see it."

Robert instructed him, "Keep thy hands perfectly relaxed. I shall now teach thee something that my uncle taught me when I was a young lad." When Thomas became perfectly relaxed, his uncle took both of Thomas' hands and put his hands directly over them. Standing behind his nephew, with Thomas' hands on the part of Dare's back that was out of alignment, Robert quickly moved his hands with force. "Dost thou feel and see what we just did?"

Thomas felt Dare's back at the point where his uncle's hands were, and noticed that Dare's back was no longer crooked, nor was there an S shape, "Yes, uncle!" he answered, amazed.

"Try to remember what we just did." Robert said. "Our dogs are working dogs. They will put their lives on the line to make sure that none of our animals get away, or are harmed. In doing so, they are prone to all kinds of injuries. There will come a time when thou may need to do alone what we have just done together." Next, Robert had his nephew roll Dare over gently on his back as he said, "Have Dare stay as still as a board, and keep him calm."

As Thomas softly spoke, "Easy mate, stay still, thou shalt be fine." Robert took his nephew's hands again, this time putting them on Dare's neck with his on top. As he had done with Dare's back, he had his nephew feel where the neck was out of alignment. This had happened at the moment that Dare collided with Bulldread in mid air.

Feeling what his uncle was talking about, Thomas asked skeptically, "Can we fix it?"

Robert took a deep breath, focused, and felt very carefully. As he had done with the back, he used just enough force on Dare's neck to cause it to pop back into place. Robert smiled as he answered, "We just did, thanks to thee for staying relaxed and keeping thy dog relaxed, too."

Thomas felt Dare's neck pop into place, he asked, "Is Dare's neck better now?"

Robert answered, "Dare's neck is a lot better; however, it is still badly sprained, as

are a lot of other muscles in his body. This dog needs a lot of love and rest for the

next several days."

Thomas replied, "What ever it takes uncle, I shall do it!

Robert then looked up, and raised his hands, praying, "I thank Thee, Lord God, for what we have been able to do so far. Now I pray Thee, help me with the hardest part." This would be Dare's shoulder, which was badly dislocated. Robert told Thomas, "Keep Dare still and calm one more time; this time it is really going to hurt." Thomas did this as his uncle very carefully felt Dare's left shoulder.

Thomas asked, "Art thou not going to place thy hands on top of mine this time?"

Robert thought about teaching his nephew this time before answering,

"This time put thy hands on top of mine and feel how we do this, and also pray silently."

Thomas put his hands on top of his uncle's hands asking, "How often have you done this before?"

Robert answered quite harshly, "Keep silent. Just pray!" Thomas prayed with his eyes closed as his uncle this time took two really big breaths. When exhaling on the second breath, he forcefully popped Dare's shoulder back into place. This caused Dare to yelp in pain. He moved his shoulder and was able to stand up for a second, but not much longer because he still had a lot of pulled muscles, along with some sprains in his neck, back, and legs. Robert sighed as he answered his nephew's question. "That, my dear nephew, was the very first time!" Robert looked into Dare's eyes. The left eye, which had been crossed, was now completely normal. Robert raised his hands up and shouted, "Halleluiah." Then he lowered his hands and grabbed Dare's face, gave him a big kiss on the cheek and said with a huge smile, "I think thou art going to survive mate, I truly do!" Robert turned to his nephew with a look of great relief. His nephew thanked him and gave him a great big hug.

Tears of joy trickled down Thomas' face, and onto his uncle's shoulder as he told him, "My greatest thanks. I do not know what I would do if me best mate were to die so young!" Afterwards, Thomas turned hugging his father, "Many thanks for getting Dare over here so fast."

"I was glad to help, son," his father replied, as he gently massaged Dare's neck with one hand and held his son with the other. "I know how much Dare means to thee. He means just as much to me as well, for I shall always remember him as the dog that saved my beloved son's life!"

Hearing this Robert asked, "What happened? How did Dare save thy life nephew?"

"Ye two better sit down. This is going to be a long story," Thomas said, rolling his eyes. He began to explain all that had happened. However, while he was explaining the part about Lord Riley, Thomas' father left the room and walked outside, away from his brother's home. He picked up a stick and began smacking it against a tree, picturing the tree as Lord Riley's head. Thomas' father couldn't handle the fact that his son had been screaming for his life, and that Lord Riley turned his head and was going to let his son lie helpless in the mud to die without lifting a bloody finger to help. This enraged Thomas' father so much that he even thought about going over to Lord Riley's manor and killing him with his own two bare hands.

After hearing the whole story, Robert remained speechless for a minute. Like his brother, he was enraged at Lord Riley, but at the same time very grateful that his favorite nephew was alive. He was astonished that Dare was able to collide with the bull in mid air and able to lock his jaws onto him so well. He was also astonished that Dare was able to kill the bull and prevent any harm from coming to his favorite nephew.

Eventually he responded, "Amazing! I have heard a lot of stories of about how our dogs have done some truly remarkable things in the past. Some of them have even saved the lives of our ancestors, like Dare saved thine. However, the story of what happened to thee today is, I must say, the most fascinating story I have ever heard." He wrapped his arms around Dare as he said, "This truly is a remarkable creature. It is a miracle he is alive right now. If he pulls through one hundred percent, which I think he will, I would really love to use him for breeding with my dogs. His genes should compliment my dogs rather nicely, if my nephew would kindly give his permission."

"Most certainly!" Thomas answered, without hesitation. "I know there will never be another dog just like Dare. However, it certainly would be nice to have a similar one."

Hearing this answer, Robert smiled as he put his hands on his nephew's shoulder.

"My thanks, nephew. That is good to hear. I will do my best to breed another Dare." Robert looked over at Dare, lying on his side injured. A happy look was upon his face as his tail wiggled slightly. Pleased, Robert told his nephew, "Stay with thy dog, give him love and keep him calm while I go speak with thy father for a while."

Robert approached his brother Justin, who was very irate, throwing rocks against a tree in the rain. "Like thee my brother, I am enraged and know exactly how thou dost feel."

"Thou hast no idea how I feel! Nor dost thou know the wrath which burns so intensely within my soul!"

"I do though my brother. After all, I love my nephew as if he were my own son! Like thee, I also feel like killing that wicked Lord Riley!"

"Let it be done then!"

"As tempting as the idea may be, we both know deep down inside that it is wrong."

"Oh, is it!" Justin replied, picking up a stick and breaking it in half against his leg. "Think thee on all the dogs' lives that we would save thus, not to mention possibly human lives!"

"I do agree with thee, my brother. We would be saving several lives. However, killing Lord Riley would still be wrong, making us just as evil as he is, and that is not what our God wants. I know it is easier said than done, but Jesus says to pray for our enemies, which is going to be exceptionally hard to do for Lord Riley."

Thomas' father interrupted, "I shall pray for him all right. I shall pray that his bloody soul burns in the pits of hell!"

"Be not consumed with anger, giving in to the desires of the Prince of Darkness, nor worry about thy son, for he is one of God's precious children. I know God has a special angel watching out for him." (At that moment, Dare struggled to raise his head up, giving Thomas a lick on the face). At this moment, Justin did not feel like hearing a sermon. He raised his voice out of anger.

"Preach not to me, my brother. Jesus also says that if anyone tries to hurt, or cause one of my little ones to stumble, it would have been better for that person if he were to have a noose tied around his throat and dropped to the bottom of the ocean. That is how Lord Riley will feel when he gets a taste of my wrath!"

Robert sighed, thinking this is going to be harder than he had thought. "That is true. But remember, the Bible says, "vengeance is mine sayeth the Lord." I promise thee, my brother, that unless Lord Riley destroys his wicked way of thinking, he shall some day suffer the wrath of our God, and that is a very dreadful thing." Robert bent down to pick up half of a large cow bone that had been given to Dare in the past. He held the piece of bone and looked at it as he said, "As I said, brother, thy son has a very special angel watching out for him. Keep in mind, thy son will never set foot on Lord Riley's estate again. Therefore, that wicked Lord Riley will no longer be a threat to him. If thou dost go forth and give in to the temptation of killing Lord Riley, more bad will come of it than good."

"With blood-thirsty eyes, Justin stared into the eyes of his brother Robert. "The evil that has manifested in Lord Riley's mind must be stopped, at any cost!"

Robert was troubled, for he saw clearly in his brother's eyes the burning desire for the spilled blood of the wicked Lord Riley. He grabbed his brother with both hands on his shoulders as he yelled in his face, "Hear what I say! Thou hast so much to lose, 'lest thou dost destroy the wicked seed of vengeance which doth grow so rapidly in your soul, else thou shalt surely turn thy precious son into an orphan! For thou shalt be hanged, surely! Thy lovely wife will be in mourning and in misery every day for the rest of her life!" A look of pain filled Robert's eyes as he continued his warning in a softer tone. "Trust me, I know. Dost thou not think that one hour hath past, in which I do not grieve for the life of my beloved wife? Words cannot express my burning desire to embrace her. This is the kind of pain that will be bestowed upon the people thou dost love."

The wicked impulses that had been sprouting within Justin died back after he heard this. He turned, shedding a few healing tears as he hugged his brother. "I do know that what thou hast said is right. It is hard though, my brother, to not kill someone who would have found it amusing to watch a bull kill my son."

Robert nodded his head replying, "I know it is! However, thou must relinquish it, for God will deal with that wicked Lord Riley someday, in His way and time."

Thomas' father closed his eyes, taking deep breaths to calm down. "I know in my heart that the time is not far when Lord Riley will kill someone. It is so hard for me to do nothing and allow this to happen."

Robert cupped his hand over the back of his brother's head as he hugged him. "Trust in God, and everything will always work out for what is best in the end."

Justin backed away from his brother with his head down. "Thou dost speak what is proper. I will not kill the evil Lord Riley, although my heart is torn, for I do fear that someday I will regret that I did not do so."

Thomas' uncle sighed with great relief. "Thou dost not know how great is my relief to hear thee say this. 'Tis certain thy decision is right, my brother. If Lord Riley does not repent, God will deal with Lord Riley in His way and time." Then Thomas' father and uncle walked inside to check on Dare. Thomas had his arms wrapped around him, crying as he prayed.

He looked up at his father and uncle with fear on his face, saying, "I have never seen a dog look more ill or injured. Pray tell me uncle, do you truly believe that my dog will be alright?"

Robert answered, "Dare's strength far exceeds that of other dogs, and he is the luckiest creature in the world to be alive right now. 'Tis a miracle in itself that he did not even break a bone! To answer the question, yes, I do believe Dare will be fine. He just needs some time to heal and recover his strength. I do believe that it would be best if Dare is not moved for a while, and stays here, so I can keep a constant eye on him."

Thomas looked up at his father, "Would my father please grant permission for me to remain here until Dare gets better?"

"Permission granted," his father answered without hesitation.

The next morning, the storm was over and the sun was shining. Charles told Emily and Sara what had happened to Thomas and Dare, and said he was on his way to Thomas' to see how they were doing. Emily was really frightened by the news. She insisted that they come along, and led the way running. Charles and Sara could barely keep up with her. When they arrived at Thomas' home, his father was outside cutting wood with an ax. Emily was the first to approach him.

"How is Master Thomas?" she asked, gasping for air.

Mr. Gentry put down his ax as he answered. "My son has a badly sprained ankle, but he shall be fine in time. Dare has some bad sprains and pulled muscles. But thanks to my brother, in time he should be fine as well. Thomas and Dare are at my brother's house right now, and will probably remain there for the next few days. If ye want to see them, I am sure Thomas and Dare would love it if the three of ye paid them a visit."

Emily thanked Thomas' father for the information and said, "I do surely hope they get better." She looked at her sister and Charles as she said, "Let us not tarry, but go at once to Robert's home." Emily led the way, running again with Sara close behind her. Charles moaned, still gasping for air as he looked at Thomas' father.

"Those young ladies have more energy than any of your brothers' dogs," Charles said just before running again. Thomas's father laughed, and cupped his hands around his mouth, shouting, "That may be so, Master Charles, but thank God they sure do not look like any of my brother's dogs! If I were your age, Charles, I would keep up with them and run right by their side."

Charles smiled as he turned, acknowledging the suggestion, then looked ahead. He was fifteen years old and his male hormones were just starting to run rampant. He admired the beauty of the girls' long hair in the breeze as they ran and he noticed the perfect curves of their bodies. Charles suddenly got his second wind and caught up with Emily and Sara in no time. Justin shook his head, laughing as he watched Charles catch up with the girls. *"Oh, yes,"* he thought. *"I remember being that age. If only I could be young again."* Justin then continued to chop wood. The three soon arrived at Thomas' uncles house. Just before they arrived, Robert's dogs barked as always, letting their master know that someone was near. Hearing this, Robert whispered putting his finger to his lips, "SHH! Good dogs, my thanks for letting me know that someone approaches. Now please stop barking. I do not wish to disturb the young master and Dare. They need rest to recover." The dogs stopped barking and walked outside with Robert to see who was approaching. When he found out that it was Thomas' friends his uncle told them, "Welcome again. Ye probably came by to ask about my nephew and Dare."

"How are our friends doing?" Charles asked, bent over with his hands on his knees, this time really gasping for air.

"They both are doing exceptionally well, considering that they tangled with an enormous bull. Let us go look in on them. They slept in my guest cottage last night." Thomas' uncle quietly walked into the cottage first, with his finger to his lips, signaling three of his dogs that were in the cottage to keep quiet. Robert had them sleep there last night, keeping watch over Thomas and

Dare. As the group walked in, they saw Thomas and Dare sleeping. Thomas was snuggled up close to his dog with his arms around him, making sure he didn't get cold. Emily thought this was the cutest thing she had ever seen. At that moment, she wanted Thomas to be her boyfriend.

Emily whispered, with a big smile, "Ah what a precious sight," before tiptoeing over. At first, she was going to give Thomas a kiss on the cheek, but thought, *"He might wake up, and maybe perhaps he does not feel the same way towards me. I do not want to embarrass myself."* So instead Emily gave Dare a little kiss on the head. Thomas started to awake that moment. He blinked his eyes and saw Emily for a fraction of a second out of the corner of his right eye. He closed them with a smile, thinking that he was still asleep and was about to have a wonderful dream about the girl of his dreams. A second latter, he realized that he wasn't sleeping, and that Emily was in fact really there. He opened his eyes really fast and wide, only to see Emily's beautiful smiling face in front of his.

"Good morning Thomas," She said, "We are sorry to hear what happened to you and Dare yesterday. How are ye two feeling now?"

Thomas felt his ankle and it was still badly sprained. "I shall be fine, my lady." He answered, "I am not concerned about myself." Turning towards Dare and gently rubbing his neck, he said, "My only concern is that of me best mate." With a tear in his eye, he looked up sadly at his uncle, speaking softly. "This is the first time that I have awakened before Dare, and not seen his face above mine, with his tongue licking me and his tail wagging."

All eyes in the room, including Robert's dogs, looked sadly at Dare, who was black and blue with large swollen bruises. Thomas started to quietly cry along with Emily and Sara.

Thomas' uncle put his finger up to his lips again, quietly responding, "Be not dismayed. Dare is surrounded by a lot of love right now. This will help him heal. His body is injured and is resting, trying to repair itself. The best thing we can do is keep praying and loving him while letting him sleep."

# CHAPTER XVII
# POWER OF LOVE

A few minutes later, Thomas used the stick that Charles had found for him. He rose to his feet, and walked outside away from Dare as his uncle followed. Thomas began to cry louder. "'Tis my fault! If I had only obeyed my father and had not crossed through Lord Riley's field, none of this would have happened! Even Dare tried to warn me not to cross!"

Thomas' father and mother had arrived seconds before, and overheard what their son had said. Mrs. Gentry hugged him as his father said, "Son, do not blame thyself for what happened. I know thou wouldst not have crossed through Lord Riley's field had the way not been clear." Thomas' father closed his eyes, and held his tongue, grinding his teeth, because he knew that Lord Riley was the cause of what had happened. He wanted to curse his name some more. However, he knew it was not the right thing to do, especially in front of his son. So he took a deep breath and calmed down a little before continuing, "Thou didst not have a way to know that Lord Riley was such an evil, heartless person, and that would turn his back on man and beast, as he did you and Dare."

"That still is not an excuse for my defiance to you, father."

"Remember son, no one is perfect. I know thou hast learned from what has happened"

"Yes, but perhaps at the cost of damaging me dog for life. This guilt would not be easy to bear!"

"Hear me my son! Fret not, nor lose faith. Thine uncle doth believe Dare will recover. Several times, I have witnessed his healing hands upon God's most loving creatures. He knows how to help them heal and I know Dare shall heal, for no creature has had more love and prayers directed towards them!"

"Thy father speaks the truth." Thomas' mother added.

Robert put his hand on Thomas' shoulder. "I do believe most strongly, now more than ever, that Dare shall recover fully. It is natural for his bruises to swell overnight as they did. He is very lucky that it was cold yesterday, for the cold helped reduce his swelling. I have listened to his heartbeat this morning, and it sounds like that of a lion!" Robert said with a smile on his face. Thomas' family and friends all gathered around him, continuing to give him words of encouragement. Thomas' faith was soon restored. He dried his tears and thanked everybody, as he turned back to his dog. He got down on his knees, placing his hands on the back of his dog's head, as he softly petted the animal and prayed silently. His friends and family all stayed with him, silently praying as well.

Several hours had passed. Thomas paused from praying for a moment and looked at them. He could see the fatigue in their faces, as they glanced at Dare, and continued to pray silently. He realized they must be hungry. Thomas knew that they had many important chores that needed attention it would be selfish of him to prevent them from attending to their business. So quietly he said, "I am very grateful for all your prayers and support. However, I think 'tis time for me to be alone with my dog."

"Art thou certain?" asked his mother.

"Yes, quite certain."

"In that case, we will honor thy request. But why not rest a little with us, son, and allow me to fix thee something to eat?"

"My thanks, but no, mother. Until my dog eats, nether shall I."

His mother looked concerned. "So be it, my son. If thou art in need of anything, pray do not forget that all here are ready to help."

"Many thanks. I do know that. Everyone here has proven friendship and loyalty towards me, far beyond measure, for which I am most grateful." Thomas paused, keeping himself from crying, before adding, "All of you have important things to attend to after you eat. I want you to address them and not be troubled about us, for we shall be fine."

With that note, they all said their good byes to Thomas, and gave Dare soft little kisses on his head, so as not to disturb him. Robert's dogs remained right by Thomas' side. Sadly, they looked on at their friend. Thomas gently put his arm around Dare, whispering quietly in his ear as a few tears trickled on his face. "See how much thou art loved, and not just by me. Thou must come back! Dost thou hear me? Thou must come back!" After several more hours had passed, Thomas eventually fell asleep as he prayed. His uncle walked in to check on Thomas and his dog, and found them sleeping, Thomas with his arm around Dare. His uncle's dogs were snuggled up close to them. Robert quietly fed his dogs and instructed them to leave some food and milk on the floor next to Dare, in case he woke up in the night and was hungry. Robert said a little silent prayer for Dare and his nephew, before giving them both a kiss goodnight on their heads.

Robert hugged his dogs just before he left, whispering, "Ye are all good dogs. Keep watching over them." The next morning soon came. Thomas was awakened from a deep sleep by wagging tails smacking against his body. He opened his eyes and was welcomed to the new morning by Dare's tongue, which gave a thorough face wash, including licking the sleepy dust out of his eyes. With a huge smile, Thomas wrapped his arms around his dog.

"Welcome back mate! I knew thou wouldst not leave me." Thomas said as he cried tears of joy, which Dare licked off his face. The other dogs that belonged to Thomas' uncle barked as they continued smacking Thomas with their wagging tails. His uncle, hearing his dogs barking, came running in the room half dressed with a concerned look on his face, which was replaced by a huge smile when he saw Dare up and lively again. Robert was greatly pleased to see this, and also pleased to see that the small amount of food that had been left for Dare had been eaten during the night.

Thomas looked up at his uncle saying, "My thanks," with a wet, slobbery face.

"Pray, do not thank me," Robert replied, not taking any credit for himself. "Give thanks to God for creating Dare with the world's strongest neck."

"I already have, uncle!"

"Good lad. Now would anybody like something to eat?"

Thomas' eyes opened up wide as he answered, "Certainly."

Dare barked loudly, which meant, "My master took the words right out of my mouth." On the way to the breakfast table, Robert looked shocked to see Dare trotting so well, and how much the swelling of his bruises had gone down.

Robert said grace over breakfast, giving special thanks to God for his healing power. They then ate pork, eggs, and oatmeal. Thomas never ate more in his whole life. Afterwards his parents and friends soon came over; they were extremely surprised and happy seeing Thomas and Dare outside playing fetch the stick together.

"I do not believe me eyes! Dare is back from the dead!" After Charles said this, they all gathered around Dare, taking turns patting and hugging him, with big smiles on their faces. Dare stood there wiggling his tail back and forth like a whip.

# CHAPTER XVIII
# LEGENDARY BULLDOG STORY SPREADS

Lord Riley told a few people a carefully edited fraction of the story of how Dare came to his master's rescue, killing Bulldread because Thomas was injured in his field and could not move. Of course, Lord Riley lied to avoid making himself look like the demented person he really was, so he told people, "Fortunately, I arrived seconds before Dare and Bulldread started to fight; otherwise, I would have instantly come to Thomas' rescue." Charles told the youngsters of the town everything that he had seen happen between Dare and Bulldread. Those young people relayed to their parents what Charles had told them. Over the next few days, stories about how Dare had killed Bulldread spread faster than gangrene. Everyone who had heard these stories and then saw Dare suddenly thought he was the best looking dog on the face of the planet, the standard by which all other dogs should be judged. Because of this, everyone suddenly now wanted to be friends with Thomas and Dare. Wherever Thomas took Dare, people complimented the dog, telling Thomas things like, "If ever you breed your dog, I would love to purchase one of his pups." This was true even of people who in the past had told Thomas that his dog was ugly and should be castrated so as to prevent him from sowing his seed, and other such hurtful comments. This really bothered Thomas, even though the people who said these things repeatedly apologized to him, and to Dare, for their cruel comments. However, Thomas knew that the only reason everyone had a sudden change of heart about his dog was that Dare had killed Bulldread. People now knew that Dare had extraordinary fighting skills, which is why people wanted a puppy sired by Dare. It wasn't because of Dare's kind, gentle loving eyes and heart; it was because they wanted power and status. Thomas knew that this was why people had a sudden change of heart about being friends with him and with Dare. Thomas was casual towards everyone, but kept his distance and never got close to anyone except Charles, Emily and Sara, because they had proven their friendship towards him. Over the next several days, their friendship continued to grow. Thomas knew that some day Dare would be bred and have wonderful pups. If people other than his true friends and family wanted one of Dare's pups (if any were left over), they would have to take a test like the one his uncle had used for the last few years with prospective owners of his pups.

Unfortunately, Thomas now faced a huge problem because of the rumors being spread about Dare, thanks to Lord Riley. Dog fighters wanted to see how good a fighter Dare really was, and were willing to risk their own dog's life to find out. Strangers would approach Thomas, presenting the challenge that their dog fights Dare. Whenever this happened, Thomas walked quickly away from the challengers, saying, "No way, I shall never let my dog fight! Your dog shall have to attack me first!"

Hearing this response, dog fighters usually would not bother Thomas any further. Some of these people would flirt with the idea of giving Thomas no choice by turning their dogs loose so as to force Dare to fight. However, the last thing most dog fighters wanted was for their dogs to kill a young lad, in which case the dog fighter might be charged with murder. Dog fighters were afraid this might happen if they just let their dogs loose to attack. Because of the constant challenges that Thomas received from dog fighters, as much as possible, he began to avoid being around people when he was with Dare. The first dog fighter that really gave Thomas a big problem was Lord Draven. Lord Draven's dogs had the reputation of being the best fighting dogs around, second only to Lord Riley's. Lord Draven was extremely jealous, mostly because Lord Riley received more money for puppies than he did. Lord Draven had a lot of pride. He lied, telling himself he had the best fighting dogs, and wanted that reputation. One day, Lord Draven was on his way to a dogfight with a few friends and his best fighting dog, Buster, when he noticed Lord Riley walking into the Larksmur town bakery with his nephew, Vivian.

Seeing this, Lord Draven pointed to Lord Riley and said to his friends, "Well I'll be damned, for there is Lord Riley Braun Warne." Lord Draven rubbed his hands together with a sinister smile. "It does appear that this is me lucky day, for here is my chance to challenge Lord Riley to a dogfight."

Lord Draven's friend, Sir Alex, commented, "Lord Riley claims that he will no longer fight his dogs against other dogs, but will only fight them against bulls or bears."

Angry, Lord Draven replied, "We shall see about that! If Lord Riley denies my challenge, I shall taunt him until he becomes fighting mad, no matter how long it takes!" Lord Draven tied Buster up outside the bakery. Then he and his friends walked into the bakery and approached Lord Riley, who was shopping for bread with his nephew Vivian. Lord Draven tapped Lord Riley on the shoulder pretty hard with his finger. Startled, Lord Riley spun around to see Lord Draven's face very close to his. Lord Draven stared into Lord Riley's squinted beady eyes with his own. Lord Riley knew Lord Draven and knew exactly what he and his friends wanted.

Lord Riley asked, "What, good sir! How can I assist you?"

"Indeed." Lord Draven answered in a quietly threatening tone. "For the longest time, you have had the reputation of owning the best fighting dogs around. I now want that reputation! Therefore, I do challenge your dogs to fight my dogs to the death in the pit!"

"I would rather not," Responded Lord Riley. "I no longer pit dog against dog."

Lord Draven raised his hands close to Lord Riley's face asking," Why? Methinks 'tis because you know my dogs will defeat your own."

Lord Riley laughed, "Surely you jest! Your dogs are no challenge. In truth, the reason is that my dogs make so much more money for me by fighting bulls and bears. Besides, the dogs I own now have never been defeated by another dog. Everyone knows that your dogs are unworthy adversaries."

Vivian spoke up with a chuckling behind his voice. "Indeed, few people will come and pay money to see your pathetic dogs killed in the pit in a fight against my uncle's dogs!" These comments enraged Lord Draven! His eyes opened wide and his face turned red. He was angry, not so much because Lord Riley denied his dogs a fight, but because he was being laughed at and his dogs had been called unworthy adversaries.

With a raised voice he replied, "Oh, yes! Laugh, then, you pathetic, arrogant bloody bastards! Your dogs have never lost in the pit because they have never fought any worthy adversaries, like my dogs! In truth, you are turning down my challenge because you know, just as I do, that your dogs will be ground into a powder if put in a pit with my dogs!" Everyone around who heard this laughed, except for Lord Riley and his nephew.

Vivian responded in a calm, sarcastic tone of voice. "A powder, me uncle's dogs? If you do truly believe this ludicrous statement, you must have taken a bad mix of some sorcerer's potion. For me uncle's dogs are far superior." Everybody around who heard this chuckled and gasped, "OOOH!"

Lord Draven angrily replied, "So you say, little bastard! In that case, why does your uncle not prove it? I shall tell you why! Because he secretly knows that his dogs will be torn apart!" Lord Riley did not like his nephew being called a bastard. He was now angry, and thought, *"Unfortunately, this imbecile is putting me in a situation in which I will have to have one of my dogs kill his. I do not want to do this. Not only will I not make any money from this fight, but one of my dogs might be injured, and be unable to fight a bull again, which is where the real money is for me."* Just when Lord Riley was about to accept Lord Draven's offer and go to get one of his dogs to fight Buster, he saw Thomas walking with Dare. They were on their way to the town's bakery to shop. Seeing this, Lord Riley quickly came up with a brilliant solution to get himself off the hook and avoid having one of his dogs fight Lord Draven's dogs.

Lord Riley pointed at Thomas and Dare as he said, "Lord Draven, look you at that dog with the lad coming our way."

Lord Draven turned looking answering, "Yes, I do see, but what about him?"

Lord Riley with a devious smile answered, "'Tis Dare, a dog that I bred; you probably have heard of him by now."

Skeptical, Lord Draven answered, "Oh yes, 'tis the dog that is said to have killed Bulldread all by himself." Lord Draven didn't believe this, because Bulldread had once killed five of his best fighting dogs at the same time.

Lord Riley nodded his head yes. "'Tis true; I did witness it myself." Lord Riley's devious smile became even wider as he said, "I shall accept your challenge that our dogs fight, on one condition."

"Name it!" Lord Draven responded intensely.

"First, your dog must defeat Dare!" Lord Riley firmly stated. "Then, and only then, shall your challenge be met." Lord Draven looked back at Thomas, who was smiling and throwing a stick as Dare fetched it with his tail wiggling back and forth.

Seeing this, Lord Draven replied, "That will be no problem. That dog is much too happy to be a fighting dog. My dog Buster is also much bigger!" With a cynical smile on his face, Lord Draven turned to Lord Riley and said, "Prepare one of your dogs to fight the best fighting dog he has ever faced in his life."

Smiling, Lord Riley replied, "If you say so. Do remember, first your fighting dog must defeat Dare." Lord Riley then paid for his bread and walked out of the bakery with his nephew before Thomas saw him. Lord Riley and his nephew slid around a corner to watch what would happen. Lord Riley didn't want Thomas to see him, fearing that Thomas would embarrass him and make his reputation even worse by yelling at him in front of everyone in the bakery or asking, "Why did you watch your bull try to kill me without trying to stop him and help me?"

As Thomas walked up to the bakery with Dare, Buster began barking at them. Thomas thought Buster was securely tied up, so he wasn't worried that while he was shopping in the bakery, Buster would get free and attack Dare. As he walked in the bakery, Thomas told Dare, "Stay, and be good, as is usual for thee. I shall return shortly." Buster looked over at Dare. He continued to bark and tried to break free from his rope so he could attack. On the other hand, Dare remained calmly laying down untied, looking at Buster with no fear in his eyes whatsoever. He thought, *"Do not tell me that you would even consider attacking me, you stupid dog. I killed a bull ten times bigger than you! I could tear you apart faster than you could take your next breath."*

Buster made eye contact with Dare, and could tell that Dare wasn't frightened or intimidated by him in any way. This made Buster even more furious at Dare. He desperately kept trying to get free so he could attack.

While this was happening, two young girls walked towards the bakery. They were afraid of Buster and walked closer to Dare. One of the girls made eye contact with Dare, and saw his kind, gentle eyes in his wrinkled face, and his tail wiggling slightly, back and forth. The young girl was not afraid. She fearlessly approached Dare as he stood up, wiggling his tail and body back and forth out of joy as the young girl approached. With a huge smile, the young girl wrapped her arms around Dare and was soon joined by her friend.

Dare licked the girls' faces as the girl who had approached Dare first laughed and said, "What a wonderful dog."

"Indeed," the other girl said as she pointed at Buster, who was growling, "Not like that mean, bloody son of a bitch!"

As Thomas walked to the rear of the bakery, Lord Draven walked over to the shop owner and handed him a half a pound, saying, "I will pay for whatever that young lad desires, and also give him the change that is left over." Lord Draven then walked outside to wait for Thomas. On his way out, Thomas passed the two girls as they went in the store. As Lord Draven made eye contact with Dare, Dare arose again to his feet. This time he quietly growled, with his ears standing up. For Dare saw through Lord Draven's soul and knew the evil which lurked within. Lord Draven walked over to Buster, who was still trying desperately to get free so he could attack. He was only a few seconds away from ripping his leash in two, when Lord Draven ordered him to shut up and lie down. Buster instantly obeyed his master.

Lord Draven looked over at Dare again, this time with a cocky expression as he said sarcastically, "So! Thou art the incredible fighting dog that is the subject of everyone's conversation." Lord Draven chuckled slightly as he said, "Surely they jest. Buster shall soon tear thee apart!"

As Thomas walked around the bakery, he noticed out of the corner of his eye, that everyone was looking at him. Thomas quickly grabbed his bread and pastry and then went to pay for them. As he did the shop owner waved up his hands, saying, " No, young master, 'tis not proper that thou purchase anything here today!"

Thomas was shocked to hear this. "Why not?" he asked, confused. "I have done nothing wrong."

The shop owner, as did everyone who was there chuckled. "Do not fret, young master," the shop owner answered as he handed Thomas a shilling. Then he pointed outside at Lord Draven, who was smiling and waving his hand at Thomas. "Look thou, dost thou see that kind Lord waving at thee?"

"Yes." Thomas answered confused.

"Well, his lordship was kind enough to pay for thy family's food today." With a stunned look on his face, Thomas gazed at Lord Draven, grabbed his food, and walked outside. Lord Draven quickly approached him with a huge smile and extended hand. Seeing this, Dare stood up and growled at Lord Draven, for he did not like this evil man anywhere near his beloved master.

Bewildered, Thomas shook Lord Draven's hand. "My thanks for the food, kind lord. Pray forgive me, but do I know you?"

Lord Draven kept smiling as he answered. "No, thou dost not. However, thou and thy dog soon will." At that moment, Buster began to go crazy again, trying even harder to get free so he could attack Dare. Lord Draven turned and looked at Buster with a mean glare and a raised right hand, which meant be quiet right now or you shall receive a severe beating. Seeing this, Buster quit barking and instantly lay down. With a smile on his face, Lord Draven turned back to Thomas. "I, young master, am a very wealthy Lord with a plan about how thou canst become wealthy, too. Wouldst thou like to hear it?"

Thomas looked over at Buster and could tell by the way he was snarling loudly and foaming at the mouth that he was restraining himself from firing up again. Thomas heard Dare's quiet growls and saw the disturbed look in his eyes, due to Buster and Lord Draven.

"Do not fret, mate," Thomas told Dare, sensing Lord Draven's evil intentions. "I shall never let any more harm come to thee ever." Thomas turned, and looking Lord Draven straight in the eyes, said, "No, my Lord, I do not wish to hear what you have in mind." After giving a firm answer, Thomas immediately turned and walked away with Dare.

Seeing this, Lord Draven shouted at Thomas, as he followed him, along with a crowd of people. "Might thou not wait a moment, you ungrateful little lad? I just handed yon merchant half a pound for thy groceries! Therefore, I insist that thou dost hear what I say!"

Thomas stopped and pulled from his pocket the money, which the shop owner had returned to him, and put it on the ground along with his groceries, as he replied, "Here, take your money and your food! I do not want either!" Thomas turned around and started to walk away again. However, this time Lord Draven's friends stood in front of Thomas and Dare, blocking their path, looking tough and mean with their arms folded.

A friend of Lord Draven named Neal said to Thomas, "You have insulted me mate by refusing his money. You shall indeed listen what he has to say, before you walk away!"

Dare didn't appreciate Neil's tone of voice towards his master. As a result, Dare gave Neal and all of Lord Draven's friends the evil eye. His lips curled back as he exposed his massive fangs, giving one of his loud and furious growls as if to say, "Move aside or your suffering will be legendary!" Seeing this, Neal and Lord Draven's friends instantly cleared the path for Thomas and Dare.

However, Thomas turned back to Lord Draven, because Thomas knew he had something on his mind that he desperately wanted to say. Thomas knew that if he didn't confront Lord Draven now, he would have to do so later. Thomas wasn't one who liked unresolved issues. So, with closed eyes, knowing he wasn't going to like what Lord Draven was about to say, he said, "Alright. Let us get this over with. What is it that you wish to tell me?"

Lord Draven answered, pointing his finger at Dare, "Your incredible beast killed Bulldread all by himself. Thanks to our good mate Lord Riley, every one now knows about it." Thomas frowned and Dare growled, hearing Lord Riley's name. His eyes remained locked onto Lord Draven's.

"Easy, mate." Thomas whispered to Dare.

Lord Draven began pacing back and forth dramatically in front of Thomas and Dare, waving his hands in the air as he spoke. "Thy magnificent beast has the reputation as the best fighting dog around. Therefore, many people will pay much money to watch him fight against others in the pit. If 'tis indeed true that your dog killed Bulldread all by himself," (Lord Draven immediately gave a slight chuckle after this remark, as if unconvinced.) "Well then, I am certain that he shall have no problem defeating any of my dogs in the pit. For there is not a bloody chance in hell any of my dogs could kill Bulldread. I assure thee, thy wonderful beast will be all right afterwards. I offer thee the chance to be the richest lad in town. All thou needst do is to let thy dog fight one of my dogs in the pit. I will arrange and promote the fight all by myself. Thou wilt not have to do a bloody thing. After the fight, I will split the money made with thee, sixty-forty."

Thomas listened with fists clenched and eyes closed very tight the whole time. Dare was also greatly disturbed, and his hair stood straight up. He knew Lord Draven had upset his master, and whenever his master was upset, he was upset. Thomas looked at Lord Draven with narrowed eyes as he breathed very heavily through flared nostrils. His teeth were closed, with lips barely open as he mumbled with a slight sarcastic tone of voice. "I know a better way for my dog to make us a lot more money, other than fighting your dog in the pit. Would you care to hear?"

"Of course I would! I am very anxious to hear it!" Lord Draven answered enthusiastically, unaware of Thomas' sarcasm. Lord Draven thought Thomas might just be starting to have a change of heart about using Dare to fight. Thomas took another deep breath before he exploded, yelling, "You fight my dog in the pit! You can even keep all the money from the event! I guarantee people would pay much more money to see this, although you would not be able to spend any of it, due to your bloody bottom being torn into a thousand pieces!" Thomas paused with a disgusted look, before saying, "People like you make me sick! You take God's most loyal creature, who will do anything it can to please its master, and turn that good creature into a mirror of your sick, bloodthirsty self! My answer is no! And it shall always be no when it comes to dog fighting!"

The nearby crowd chuckled at Lord Draven, (with the exception of his friends) and made comments like, "That young lad certainly told him," and, "Indeed, I would pay a lot of money to see a dog fight a dogfighter!"

This made Lord Draven furious. "So be it, little bastard!" he responded out of rage. "'Tis a bloody shame thou dost refuse my offer to have Dare fight in the pit against my dog. For thou wouldst be guaranteed easy money, an amount of money for which most people sweat blood for years."

"Your name should be Judas, for you sell unconditional love towards thyself for blood money."

"Call it what thou dost wish, young fool; my money works just as well as any hard working person's money."

"How can you sleep at night if you think like that?"

"I do sleep much easier than if I had to sweat blood all day making someone else a rich Lord." (Hearing Lord Draven's comments, the crowd looked at him with animosity, for they themselves were hard workers.) "Now, because of your foolishness, I shall untie Buster, and thus your dog shall be forced to fight."

"Stop!" Thomas said, standing directly in front of Dare, as Lord Draven walked towards Buster, "For you have nothing to gain if your dog fights us."

"Oh! But I do!" Lord Draven stopped, turned and replied. "For in doing so, I shall prove to everyone here, by the victory that is soon to be Buster's, that he is a worthy adversary for any of Lord Riley's fighting dogs!" Lord Draven turned, continuing towards Buster as he warned, "I strongly advise moving away from your beast's side!"

"Never! Your dog shall have to kill me first!"

Lord Draven paused and thought, *"He is bluffing. Surely he will flee, once he sees a real fighting dog charge towards him!"* Without turning around, he replied, "So be it," then continued walking.

Hearing this, the crowd was awed, and Lord Draven's friends gulped as they exchanged worried glances. Someone in the crowd spoke up. "Lord Draven's gone mad."

Lord Draven clapped his hands twice as he approached Buster, a signal that meant get ready dog, you are about to be in a fight to the death. Buster responded by going crazy, pacing back and forth while staring in Dare's eyes, and was ready to attack.

As Lord Draven reached out to untie Buster, Thomas yelled again at him. "If you let your dog loose, I shall kill you!"

As he was about to untie Buster and let him go, Lord Draven turned again to look at Thomas. "Do not be absurd, little bastard!" he said with a sinister chuckle. "You're not even half my size. You do not have a prayer of killing me."

As Lord Draven started to untie Buster, Thomas replied, "What you say is true, Sir. However, my dog can kill you easily! Therefore, before you release your dog, sir, you had better be bloody sure he is able to kill my dog! For if he does not and my dog sees you hurting me, he shall turn to you and bite your face off! And he will do much worse to you than he did to Bulldread when he tried to attack me! If that happens, I promise, you shall surely die a bloody and painful death!"

Lord Draven looked at Dare just as he was about to finish untying Buster. Dare knew that Buster was almost untied. It didn't take Dare more than a second to go into killing mode. He jumped in the air, doing a complete three sixty, running towards Buster with exposed massive jaws that were razor sharp. He gave an unheard of loud barking growl, which caused chills to streak through everyone's spine, including Busters. Seeing Dare in killing mode, Lord Draven became petrified.

With shaking hands, he quickly tied Buster back up securely as he told Thomas, "Call your dog off! Perhaps I will talk you into fighting Dare some other time."

Thomas whistled to Dare, "Come here mate; let us go home," (as he gave Lord Draven the evil-eye.) Dare instantly snapped out of killing mode, wagging his tail, and becoming his peaceful self again. Thomas walked away with Dare, keeping a mean glare on Lord Draven as he warned. "Never again force your dog upon mine and never again speak to me about dog fighting." Lord Draven gulped with fear and made damn sure Thomas and Dare were a long distance away before he untied Buster. The people around looked at Lord Draven and shook their heads thinking, *"You have the courage to talk, but are a coward when it comes to action."*

Seeing the people shaking their heads, Lord Draven responded defensively, "I say! What do ye expect me to do? Kill a child!" Hearing this, the people laughed, for everyone knew that this was just an excuse and that Lord Draven was afraid for his life, and rightfully so.

Lord Riley had watched the whole thing with his nephew from a short distance away. The two had been greatly entertained. Lord Riley figured that there was no way Thomas would fight Dare for money. Otherwise, he would have made Thomas an offer to set up fights himself, and would have paid Thomas twice as much money as Lord Draven.

Lord Riley's nephew Vivian was in awe about how fast Dare could transform himself from a fun loving, tail-wagging dog, into a fanged, snarling killer. Vivian turned to his uncle and asked, "Do you believe that Dare is the best fighting dog?"

Lord Riley answered, "Never have I witnessed a dog attacking with more power and agility than Dare. There is only one dog who would be a worthy adversary for Dare."

"Who?" Vivian eagerly interrupted, hoping that his uncle would say his dog's name in answer.

"His brother, Terror." Lord Riley paused in awe at the thought of the two brothers fighting someday, and then continued, "I guarantee, that would be the best bloody dogfight in history."

Vivian's pride crept into the picture. He thought that his dog Angus was the best fighting dog, so he asked, "Might my dog Angus also be a worthy adversary?"

Knowing what the outcome would be, Lord Riley responded with a slight chuckle, then answered, "No!"

"What if we trained Angus to kill better?"

"His training would be in vain if matched against Dare." After answering, Lord Riley came to an abrupt stop with a sigh of frustration, knowing his nephew's determined intentions. He stared in Vivian's eyes as he lectured him. "Dare, like his brother, is an accident, a freak of nature. Until now, thou hast had the best fighting dog any young lad has owned. I know it must be hard to know that someone else has a dog superior to thine. Luckily for me, that is a situation which I never had to endure." Hearing this, Vivian became angry. His mouth grimaced as he closed his eyes and took a deep breath. "The look thou just gave when hearing what I just said reveals thou art angry," Lord Riley continued to walk and talk, trying to make his nephew feel better. "Heed my words. Someday thou shalt own a dog capable of defeating all his foes, including Terror and Dare."

Vivian didn't feel any better. He didn't want to wait for a dog capable of defeating all his foes. He tried defending Angus again, saying, "Angus has never suffered defeat. What makes you so certain that he could not defeat Dare? After all, you did never imagine that Dare would amount to anything and did leave him in the forest to die!"

Annoyed, Lord Riley responded, "Leaving Dare in the forest was the biggest mistake I ever made. I used to think size matters and was terribly mistaken."

Vivian interrupted, "Might there be a chance that you are wrong about Angus?"

"Not a bloody chance in hell!" Lord Riley answered harshly.

"Remember at the last bull baiting event how Angus and a few of his brothers destroyed a bull."

"Indeed I do," Lord Riley answered, concerned about his nephew's pride. "With the help of four of his brothers, Angus devoured the bull, for they all worked well together as a team. Dare, on the other hand, devoured a bull all by himself! I do assure thee, 'twould be impossible for Angus to kill a healthy bull by himself, let alone kill Dare!" A few seconds of uncomfortable silence passed before Lord Riley continued, "I know what thou dost think, but let that thought go. For if thou dost put Dare to the test, Angus will be devoured! And thou shalt be humiliated"

Vivian pondered his uncle's comments for a minute before asking, "Remember Uncle, the time when you did tell me that your dogs are also mine?"

"Yes, I remember."

"In that case, may I borrow Terror and prove to me mates that I still have the best fighting dog?"

Lord Riley was taken off guard by this trick question. Enraged, Lord Riley stopped abruptly and grabbed his nephew's shoulders near his throat. "Perish that thought!" He said with a furious tone. "If ever thou dost think to borrow Terror to fight, I do swear I shall choke thee to death with my own bare hands! Nobody fights Terror but me, for I will make more money from him than from all our other dogs combined!" After saying this, he calmed down, giving a quick chuckle as he released his hands. "Besides, Terror is the most ferocious beast in the world. Wouldst thou ever be fool enough to try to borrow him, he would tear thee to pieces before thou hast left my yard." Vivian continued to walk with his uncle, with his head held slightly down. His pride was very hurt. Until now, no lad his age ever had half as good a fighting dog as Angus. This situation was hard for Vivian to accept.

# CHAPTER XIX
# PRIDE GOETH BEFORE A FALL

Thomas patted Dare on the head on their way home, saying, "If anyone troubles thee, they trouble me as well." Dare felt his master's love towards him. With a wagging tail, Dare tackled his master, knocked him to the ground, and wrestled with him, tickling and soaking him with his tongue. A few seconds later, he pinned his master by gently putting his teeth on top of his master's nose, making sure, as always, not to injure him. With his nose pinned, Thomas mumbled, "Release me at once, thou crazed beast!" A minute later he was released. Shaking his head, Thomas rose to his feet in disgust. He brushed off all the dirt from his clothes with his hands, while giving his dog the evil eye. "Many thanks!" he said sarcastically. "Shouldst thou ever do that again, thy suffering shall be legendary." Dare had heard these words over a hundred times before, and knew that his master was not serious. He wagged his tail as the two continued to walk home.

Word immediately spread about Thomas and Dare's encounter with Lord Draven. Vivian's acquaintances had heard what had happened. They, like several other people, wanted to see just how good a fighting dog Dare really was. Henry, a tall, hefty lad, came up with a plan to praise Dare highly to Vivian, in the hope of making him madly jealous, so he would put his dog to the test. Henry discussed this idea with the rest of Vivian's acquaintances. Immediately afterward, out of the corner of his eye, Henry saw Vivian walking with Angus. "Good day, Vivian," he said to him in a sarcastic tone. "Have you heard the latest news about Dare? You know Dare, the best fighting dog around, the one that killed your uncle's bull all by himself."

With a perturbed look on his face, Vivian answered, "'Tis the freak, you do mean! What about him?"

"Lord Draven did challenge Thomas to a dog fight and would not take no for an answer. Well, that is, until Thomas made threats to release Dare upon him after the dogs fought."

Stanley chuckled, adding, "Never have I heard of anyone being as petrified as was Lord Draven upon hearing this."

Henry also chuckled, commenting, "'Twould be nice to own a dog that could fight like Dare, I say. I wager that thou wouldst love to own a dog like that, too. Do you not agree, Vivian?" Vivian's acquaintances all chuckled as Henry added sarcastically, "Just imagine having a dog capable of defeating any foe. Oh! Pray forgive me, Vivian! You did once have a dog like that!" Vivian kept quiet, remembering what his uncle had said.

Vivian's acquaintances continued, adding more derogatory comments like, "Look you, Vivian. Why not buy Dare with your uncle's money? In that way, you will once again own the best fighting dog!"

Henry added, "Perhaps you should learn what Thomas is feeding Dare. Possibly then Angus will be almost as good a fighter as Dare!" Vivian remained quiet, grinding his teeth with rage. Seeing Vivian angry, Henry did not let up. He patted Vivian on the back, continuing sarcastically, "Do not feel bad, mate. For several years, your dogs have been the best fighters; now they are not. So again I say, do not trouble yourself, for you can still reminisce about yesterdays." Vivian remained quiet, but his hands began to shake due to rage.

Stanley also patted Vivian on the back, commenting, "Do cheer up, mate! Think you back to your days of boasting that Angus was the best fighting dog. Do you remember Ashton Driscoll?"

"Certainly," Vivian answered with a sudden look of pride. "He used to boast about War's undefeated victories; that is until War faced Angus."

"'Tis right, for Ashton became tired of all your boasting that Angus was the best. Therefore, he accepted your challenge, in which Angus mercilessly proved you right." Stanley clapped his hands once, keeping them together, and smiled sarcastically before continuing. "Well mate, that was yesterday. Today, 'tis Dare who is the number one dog in town. 'Tis best that you continue to reminisce, because Angus's ruling days are gone!" This was the first time in Vivian's life that he had been mocked due to his dogs. He brushed off his shirt where Henry and Stanley's hands had touched him.

Vivian could no longer control his pride. Enraged, he yelled, "You do speak out of ignorance! 'Tis I who have always had the best fighting dog, and I still do. Angus could tear Dare apart faster than one could blink an eye!" Henry smiled in great delight, along with everyone there.

"Prove it, Vivian!" challenged Stanley, "Prove it!"

Out of rage, Vivian replied, "I shall!" as he took Angus with a determined look saying, "Let us go find that son of a bitch! For this shall be the last day of his bloody life!" Everyone around hearing this replied by yelling, "Dog fight! Dog fight!"

With smiles, Henry and Stanley, slapped one another's hands as Henry said, "We did it mate, we made him bloody fighting mad!" Henry and Stanley followed as Vivian and Angus searched for Thomas and Dare. Henry's plan to make Vivian fighting mad had worked.

As Vivian searched for Thomas and his dog, more people around heard the words "Dog fight!" so more and more people joined in, following the crowd. Soon, even more people began chanting, "Dog fight!" They searched all over town for hours. They looked for Thomas by a river, near where he often went fishing. They even searched for Thomas at the church where he and Dare often pulled weeds together for charity work, but with no luck. They even searched in the neighboring towns, but only found still more bloodthirsty people who followed along, wanting to see a free bloody dog fight to the death. Hours later, after walking several long miles, Vivian, along with now nearly a hundred bloodthirsty followers, finally ran into Thomas and Dare, who were returning from a fun day together at Thomas' uncle's house. Charles, Emily, and Sara were with them.

In a furious tone of voice, Vivian pointed at Thomas and Dare saying, "There ye are! We have been searching all over for the pair of ye. I do think that ye knew that we were looking for you and became terrified, with good reason! That is why ye cowards left town, hoping we would stop searching for ye when ye returned. But much to your dismay, we did not!" Thomas had a stunned look on his face, not knowing that Vivian and the crowd were there to see his dog fight.

"What reason would I have to be afraid of ye?" Thomas asked with open hands. Hearing that, the crowd said "OOOOH," for they thought that Thomas was mocking Vivian, and so did he.

"I shall inform you why 'tis that you do need to fear me." answered Vivian, enraged. "My dog Angus is a far superior fighter to yours. He shall prove it by tearing your has-been mongrel into a thousand pieces."

Immediately after Vivian yelled this, Henry looked around at the crowd that had followed them. With a raised hand he chanted, "ANGUS! ANGUS! ANGUS!" Henry influenced his friends and all the people around to slowly chant likewise. At that moment, Vivian heard his uncle's words going through his head again. "If thou dost put Dare to the test, he shall devour Angus and thou shalt be humiliated!" Vivian looked at Dare, and noticed the dog's rippling muscles, huge chest, and gigantic skull. Vivian didn't see an ounce of fat on him either. Starting to seriously doubt that his dog could defeat Dare, Vivian turned his back on everyone, looked down on the ground, and saw a large stone. With beady eyes, Vivian looked around to make sure that nobody could see what he was about to do. Then, very deviously and quickly, he bent over and picked up the large stone. He planned to help Angus win the fight by discreetly stoning Dare. Before this, Thomas had already had to deal with several other people who had challenged his dog to fight with their dogs. Thomas knew by the determined, bloodthirsty look in Vivian's eyes that he wasn't going to leave without a fight.

So, Thomas rolled up his sleeves, and shouted at Vivian. "I do see, by the presence of all these good people assembled here, that you no doubt did promise a fight! THEREFORE, A BLOODY FIGHT THEY SHALL SEE!" Hearing this, the crowd cheered, believing they were about to see Dare fight.

Hearing Thomas' comments, Emily became very angry with him. "I did think thee a kindhearted lad!" She scolded, "Thine uncle would be furious at thee! No one in thy family has ever fought dogs before! I am certain that some of thy departed relatives will turn over in their graves shouldst thou follow through with thy plan and fight Dare! Besides, thou didst give thy word that thou wouldst never fight dogs."

Thomas touched Emily on the shoulder, and quietly said, "Do not be fret, Emily; my word is good. I shall not break any vows!" Out of disgust, Emily quickly brushed his hand away from her. Emily had her back turned to Thomas and did not acknowledge him as he continued to speak. "In truth, I do like thee very well, my lady. However, pray do understand, I have no choice in this matter." Thomas paused for a second, thinking that if Emily were to stay, she would probably lose respect for him. "Perhaps thou might prefer to take thy leave now, because I am bloody angry, and 'twould not be proper for my lady to see this side of me. Therefore, pray take thy leave." But Emily would not leave, nor would her sister, because what Thomas had said made them want to stay all the more. Knowing that the girls were not going to leave, Thomas gave up trying, and turned to Vivian, shouting. "As I have told others, now I hereby do tell you! I shall never fight dogs for money, for pride, or for any other reason! Therefore, instead, to give the crowd what they do desire, and to shut your foolish bloody bottom up, I shall fight you! Come now, you great scalawag, let us fight!"

Hearing this, the crowd became suddenly quiet. These people had not walked for miles on end just to see two lads fight. Before this, Vivian had only fought three times in his life, and he had lost on all three occasions. He was a would-be bully who could not fight, which is one of the reasons he got into dog fighting in the first place, so he could have his dogs fight instead of himself. Vivian looked at Thomas, and was intimidated, knowing that Thomas was very angry with him. Vivian knew if they fought, he would probably be badly beaten up, which would be humiliating as well as painful. So very cleverly, to keep the crowd on his side without embarrassing himself he lied, saying, "Who are you trying to fool? You have been blinded by religion and have never fought a day in your life!" Vivian paused, smirking arrogantly. "I, on the other hand, am a fighter, and have been victorious in every fight I have encountered." (Hearing this, Henry and Stanley exchanged looks of disbelief, for they knew for a fact that Vivian was lying about this.) "All here know that you are an unworthy opponent for me. These people would prefer to see our dogs fight, because they already know that I can easily kick all the bloody shite out of you!" Hearing this, Thomas shook his head with a smile, chuckling. Annoyed with Thomas' reaction, Vivian asked, "What do you find so amusing?"

Never losing his smile, Thomas answered, "Let us hope I do not kick all the bloody shite out of you, for if I did, nothing would be left!" Hearing this, Thomas' mates laughed, along with the whole crowd, including Vivian's acquaintances. Vivian surveyed the crowd from side to side, and saw that every eye was wet with tears of laughter. Thomas had succeeded in winning the crowd over and humiliating Vivian, but more importantly, he got the crowd's thoughts distracted from the idea of Dare fighting.

After commanding Dare to stay, Thomas raised his hands and took several steps towards Vivian. He motioned with his hands for Vivian to come to him, while saying, "Come bloody swine! 'Tis time to prove how full of shite you are!"

Vivian, to avoid getting beaten up and humiliated further, very cleverly raised his hands, replying, "Let us ask the people whom they would rather see fight." Then, with a smile he addressed the crowd, asking, "Would ye rather see a little bloody fight between two lads, in which nether of us shall die?" The crowd did not respond, their thoughts were *"who cares?"* Two seconds later he shouted the question, "Or would ye rather witness a fight to the death between two beasts, with blood and guts spurting everywhere?" Upon hearing the words *blood* and *guts*, the crowd instantly cheered, chanting, "Dog fight! Dog fight!" Vivian succeeded in getting the crowd's attention back to the idea of the two dogs fighting, rather than focused on a fight between Thomas and himself. Hearing the roaring crowd, Thomas walked slowly backwards towards Dare, while keeping an eye on Vivian. When he came within a few feet of Dare, Vivian let Angus off of his leash, and pointed at Dare, commanding, "Kill"

Seeing Angus running towards his dog, Thomas commanded, "Run quickly, Dare! Do not fight!" As Angus charged, Dare stared deep into his eyes, making certain Angus was focused on him only, for if Angus had so much as glanced at his master, or any of his master's friends, Dare would have disobeyed his master's command, in which case Angus would suffer the merciless jaws of death. Luckily for Angus, he was focused on Dare. At the precise moment that Angus sprang with an open mouth, Dare spun around, avoiding being bitten. Because Dare was so focused on Angus, he didn't see that Vivian had thrown a stone at him, which was on course to hit him in the head. The whole time, Thomas was watching Vivian out of the corner of his eye, and was the only one who saw Vivian throw the stone at Dare. At the last second, to protect his dog, Thomas jumped in front of Dare's head as the stone was in the air, and was hit in the stomach. Upon being hit, Thomas crouched over, reaching out his hands, and managed to catch the stone before it hit the ground. With great will and with every fiber of his being, Thomas remained on his two feet without falling to the ground or making any noise, because he knew that if he screamed in pain, which he very badly felt like doing, his dog would stay and fight to the death for him. Thomas also knew that Dare wouldn't just be fighting Angus, but would have a second adversary in Vivian, who would be throwing a lot more stones at him. With his face slightly blue from having the wind knocked out of him, Thomas hid his intense pain, that is, until Angus followed Dare over a steep hill far away. Once the dogs were far away, Thomas collapsed on the ground in great pain, his eyes tearing, as he held his stomach and tried to catch his breath. Seeing Thomas on the ground in agony, Vivian knew that he was in no condition to fight. Therefore, Vivian took advantage of the situation. He walked towards Thomas with his hand hitting his knuckles.

With a devilish smile, Vivian said, "Your freak of nature has just proven to all assembled that he is nothing more than a coward." He paused, looking at the hill the dogs ran over, before stating arrogantly, "Heed my words! This shall be the last day you shall lay eyes on your freak of a beast, for Angus shall eventually catch Dare, and shall tear him into a bloody mess! Unfortunately, however, because of your freak's cowardly action, he has deprived everyone here of this morbid sight!" With his eyes narrowed with rage, Vivian looked back down at Thomas, and said, "I now shall attempt to satisfy the crowd's desire for blood by accepting your challenge." Vivian paused, with a quick chuckle before continuing, "So I say, rise to your feet and fight, and let us see who will have the bloody shite beaten out of him!" Thomas remained on his knees as he slowly lifted his head and glanced up at Vivian. "Well!" Vivian responded to Thomas' look. "Are you going to remain on your knees, pretending to be sick or injured to try to avoid a fight, like your cowardly freak of a beast, or will you rise and fight?"

The crowd was upset with Thomas for depriving them of their thirst for blood by telling his dog to run. They scolded him with derogatory comments like, "Rise to your feet and fight, cowardly lad! Stop holding your stomach! We all know you are neither ill nor injured!" Thomas was in great pain, but was also furious at Vivian. He attempted to rise and fight.

Charles, who was standing next to Thomas, knew that his friend was not faking. He put his hand on Thomas' shoulder, keeping him on one knee and preventing him from rising to his feet as he gave Vivian the evil eye, "Me mate is in no condition to fight! Therefore, I shall fight in his place!" Charles patted Thomas on the shoulder telling him, "Stay and rest, mate."

Knowing that Charles would defeat Vivian, Henry got involved. He put his huge hands around Charles's throat and choked him as he said, "This fight shall be between Thomas and Vivian, and nobody else, understand?" Charles tried to speak, but was unable to do so because he was being choked so hard. Just when Charles started to feel faint and his eyes started to water, he was released, surprisingly rescued by someone even bigger than Henry, namely James Tate who happened to be there with his brother Derrick. The two brothers remembered what Thomas had done for them, and they were thrilled to have a chance to repay the favor. James grabbed Henry by the throat with his left hand, and the back of Henry's left knee with his right hand, then lifted Henry over his head and threw him to the ground. He landed flat on his back, pulling several back muscles while having the wind knocked out of him. James then stood on top of Henry, and grabbed him by the throat with his left hand, then cocked his right hand back, making a fist. With a threatening tone of voice, James told Henry. "Anyone who is a friend of my brother Thomas is a friend of mine! Anyone who fights with a brother or friend of mine fights with me."

Henry was holding his back with his left hand and extending his right hand; he took a few moments to catch his breath, and then acknowledged James. "Alright," Henry gasped. "You win. I shall not fight with Thomas or any of his friends ever again. Pray, do not inflict any more pain on me."

Hearing this, James let go of Henry's collar, telling him, "You are most fortunate that there is a crowd. Otherwise, you would have been thrown to the ground headfirst, which is what will happen if Thomas or his friends are bothered again!"

Emily and Charles helped Thomas up, who wobbled over to James with an extended hand saying, "My thanks!"

James shook Thomas' hand, and pulled him to his chest, giving him a great big hug replying, "Thou art our brother. Brothers do not shake hands; they hug."

James gave Thomas a really big hug, causing Thomas to cry out, "Ouch!"

James quickly realized that Thomas' stomach was really sore and that he was hugging too hard, so he stopped with a slight chuckle, saying, "Aw, my apologies, little brother. I was unaware of my strength."

"'Tis alright, do not fret." Thomas mumbled in a hurt tone, extending his arms out to Derrick saying, "Gently, pray." Thomas then introduced James and Derrick to Charles, who was shocked to meet them, because those two lads had the reputation of being the meanest troublemakers ever.

James and Derrick shook Charles' hand, telling him, "'Tis very nice to meet you." Charles stood there speechless with his mouth open, shaking their hands. Thomas introduced Emily and Sara to James and Derrick.

James smiled as he asked Thomas, "Wouldst thou take offense if we gave the ladies an embrace?"

Thomas patted James on the back answering. "Tis alright with me, if agreeable to the ladies. But, pray do not hug them as tightly as thou didst me."

Unaware of James and Derrick's past, Emily didn't think twice about it. With a huge smile on her face and her arms extended, she responded, "Of course, 'tis alright to give us a hug." She hugged James and Derrick, and said "Our thanks, kind lads, for coming to the rescue of Thomas and Charles." Sara did the same, but was a little hesitant because she was aware of James's and Derrick's past.

James could tell by looking at the faces of Sara and Charles that they were intimidated by his brother and himself, so he said to them, "Methinks ye two are probably aware of our past."

With his arm around Thomas' neck, Derrick gave a friendly headlock. "But thanks be to our new brother Thomas, we are no longer the way we were!"

Hearing this, Sara smiled as she replied, "I am glad you have changed your ways for the better, and am very happy to be your friend."

Charles shook hands again with James and Derrick, saying, "My sentiments exactly."

Meanwhile, Vivian was surrounded by his acquaintances, and was telling them, "There are eleven of us and four of them. Therefore, I say we kick the bloody shite out of those bastards."

Moving his neck around to try to get rid of the kinks he was feeling, Henry replied without enthusiasm, "Yes, there may be eleven of us, but have you not noticed James and Derrick standing over there? They are much larger and can fight better than any of us. I would rather not tangle with either of them again!"

Vivian sighed and rolled his eyes as he replied, "Oh, pray, do not be such a coward! Yes, I notice James and Derrick standing over there. However, look you at those two, smiling and laughing with those pathetic losers! They are not the same strong and awesome lads we used to know, beating people up without reason. I believe they have turned soft and have become weaker."

Henry was still in pain from being body slammed to the ground, and with his hand on his back, he replied, "I do disagree most strongly; my back and neck prove to me that they are just as strong as they ever were!"

Vivian took a deep breath while he shook his head in disgust and said, "You just handle Charles! I will fight Thomas by myself. That means we will have nine lads against James and Derrick. Victory shall be ours!"

Henry stood up straight, feeling better because he didn't have to fight with James or Derrick again. He hit his hand against his fist saying, "'Twould surely be most agreeable to see James suffer for the pain he has caused me." He paused, smiling deviously, and said, "You are right. Victory shall be ours! Let us show James and Derrick what happens when you abandon true friends and exchange them for pathetic rabble."

"'Tis the Henry that I know and love," Vivian replied while patting him on the back. "Let us now spare no mercy on those bloody bastards."

With a phony smile, Henry nodded, thinking, *I do surely wish that Vivian did not just pat me on the back so hard: that certainly hurts.* Vivian's acquaintances turned around with angry, bloodthirsty looks on their faces as they walked towards Thomas and his friends.

Emily was the first to notice Vivian and his enraged acquaintances walking towards them. Knowing their intentions, she ran towards Vivian, as Thomas shouted at her, "No, Emily! Come back!" Thomas tried running to Emily, but due to his injured stomach, all he could do was hobble slowly. When Emily approached Vivian and his acquaintances, she stood so that Vivian couldn't come any closer without knocking her out of the way.

Emily tried reasoning with Vivian. "Me mates do not wish to fight. Why do you not go away and leave us alone?"

Vivian responded, chuckling at the thought of her stopping them. He did not wish for the crowd to hear him threaten a lady, so he mumbled quietly to Emily so the crowd couldn't hear: "Because pretty lady, I shall kick the bloody shite out of your cowardly friend, and teach Derrick and James that nobody hurts any of me mates and gets away with it! Step aside now, foolish lady, before you get hurt like your unfortunate friends are about to do."

Emily stood her ground, and did not budge. She raised her voice as she replied, so that the crowd could hear, "So be it! Hurting me is the only way you shall get past! And to think that you call me mate Thomas and his dog cowards because they do not wish to fight, when in fact you are the cowards, the proof of which is that you only fight when and if you greatly out number your opponents!" Emily paused, looking around, before challenging him, "Prove to everyone here that you are not cowardly hypocrites by making it even. Use six of your best fighters against us six."

"I have heard enough out of you!" Vivian replied out of rage, raising his open right hand. "Since you refuse to step aside, you shall now be forced!"

Vivian was just about to slap Emily when Henry very intelligently grabbed his arm. He looked around at the crowd, which was starting to look at them like they were big bad bullies. Henry whispered in Vivian's ear, "Look mate, we out number them. The last thing we need is for people in this crowd to take their side and fight against us, which is what will happen if we hurt these two ladies."

Sensing that Vivian was about to be violent with Emily, a young lady in the crowd shouted, "If you hurt her, the rest of us ladies will beat the bloody shite out of all of ye!"

Another young lady added, "We will also make bloody sure none of you shall be able to bear offspring!" Vivian and the rest of his acquaintances swallowed, cringing as they thought about what the young lady had shouted. Keeping his head still, Vivian surveyed the crowd with his eyes. He could tell by their facial expressions that the people in the crowd had no respect for him and were beginning to look like they were ready to take action against him. Vivian looked at Emily. She had closed her eyes the second Vivian had raised his hand as if to hit her. Emily kept her eyes closed, thinking, *"At any second, I shall be struck."*

With a changed and suddenly peaceful tone of voice, Vivian spoke aloud so everyone could hear. "I never had any intention of hurting this nice, lovely young lady." (Hearing this, Emily opened her eyes with surprise and said, "Hah." The first thing she saw was Vivian's hand extended, trying to shake hers. Knowing his intentions were bad, Emily backed away, avoiding letting her hand be touched.) Vivian continued, "Heavens no! I was merely trying to scare this brave young lady, to convince her to step aside so I could take Thomas up on his challenge to fight. However, she would not budge, for which I do have the greatest respect for this fearless lady. Me mates and I were not really planning to fight these lads and ladies. Heavens no! This sweet young lady was right when she stated that would make us cowards, and cowards we are not! I only wanted to strongly intimidate Thomas so that he would not back out of his own challenge and would fight me." Vivian gave the evil eye to Thomas, who was now by Emily's side, then continued, "Thomas, on the other hand, has proven here today that he is indeed a coward, for he should have instantly been by his lady's side, protecting her as she did him."

Emily knew this was not true and interrupted him with a raised voice. "Thomas would have been at my side instantly, had he not been injured!"

Vivian smiled, shaking his head back and forth, and said, "My lady continues to amaze me! Look you how she defends the cowardly bastard." Vivian began clapping loudly. "Let us hear it for this special lady, one whom I know shall never allow herself to be wooed by a bumbler such as Thomas." Vivian's acquaintances joined in whistling, chuckling, and sarcastically clapping their hands together. The crowd of people slowly joined in the clapping as well. Thomas closed his eyes, put his hands on his stomach, and took three deep breaths. His stomach felt remarkably better. Vivian laughed, thinking that he had humiliated Thomas in front of half the town, and had gotten the better of him. But much to Vivian's surprise, Thomas opened his eyes, and glared at him with a half smile as he also joined in clapping his hands together very loudly. Vivian's smile dropped as he said to Thomas, "You have just been ridiculed. For what reason are you smiling and applauding?"

Thomas took Emily's hand and kissed it softly. "I am applauding for the same reason that I do hope everyone here is clapping: for this lovely, fearless young lady." Then Thomas began to hit his fist against his hand, sarcastically saying as he walked within inches of Vivian's face, "I am certain that you are pleased to be informed that I am feeling much better now, and that I am ready to make good on my challenge." Hearing this, Vivian swallowed hard out of fear. He glanced at his acquaintances, expecting a little help from them, but much to his dismay, they had all slowly backed away from him.

Surprised and scared, Vivian looked at his acquaintances. They knew that Vivian wanted them to intervene. However, the last thing they wanted was the crowd against them. Therefore, Henry told Vivian, "Sorry mate, but like you said, it would be cowardly of us to fight people that we outnumber. You will have to fight and beat Thomas on your own." So they just stood back and watched.

Thomas shoved Vivian, saying, "Come on! You and your family force your dogs to fight! Now you fight!" Vivian trembled, and with his head held down, looked side to side. Thomas shoved Vivian even harder, causing him to go back several more feet. "Come on, you do give such a big speech about how I am a coward and you act as if you are so courageous. Aye, you are brave all right, just as long as your opponent is injured! Or else you have your dogs fight for you, because you are too much of a bloody coward to fight yourself!" Vivian kept his head down and remained unresponsive. Thomas pushed Vivian even harder, this time knocking him to the ground.

The crowd all began to laugh at Vivian, who just lay in the dirt, as his acquaintances scolded him, saying, "Come on Vivian! Get up and fight! You are making a fool out of yourself and us. Fight him, damn it!" However, Vivian did not get up and remained motionless.

Thomas walked over to Vivian and looked down at him. Shaking his head and pointing his finger near Vivian's face, Thomas said, "You are the worst, and the bloodiest excuse for a human being ever to live! You had better pray that my dog comes back alright, for if he has so much as a scar on him from defending himself, I swear to all that is holy, I shall show no mercy as I kick all the bloody shite out of you, which, as I stated before, means that there shall be nothing left of you." Hearing this and seeing Vivian cower in the dirt, the crowd began to laugh hysterically, while sarcastically using Vivian's own words against him, like, "Oh' Thomas has proven he is a coward! Unlike me mates and I!" which was followed by, "Ha! Ha! Ha!" Or, "I, unlike Thomas, am a fighter and have been victorious in every fight!" followed again by more laughter. By now, Vivian's acquaintances were really embarrassed by the crowd, and had turned their backs to the crowd to try to hide their faces. Thomas sighed, looking at Vivian in the dirt, and shook his head as he told him, "By remaining there on the ground, you have proven yourself a coward. There is no time for me to waste. Therefore, I must leave at once, find my dog, and make sure he is alright!" Thomas waved his hand at Vivian as he turned and walked away as if to say, "How pathetic." Everyone in the crowd looked at Vivian the same way. Knowing that Thomas was focused only on his dog, Vivian quickly got up and ran towards Thomas when he was not looking.

Vivian was just about to sucker punch Thomas when Emily shouted, "Behind you!" At that moment, Thomas realized what Vivian was trying to do. Thomas quickly spun around, using a move he had learned from wrestling with Dare. Quickly, he took Vivian to the ground and put him in a submissive hold. Vivian begged for mercy, as Thomas twisted his neck and arm.

Thomas told him, "Mercy shall only be shown if you give your word never again to trouble me mates, my dog, and me!" Vivian quickly gave his word, but of course his word didn't mean a thing. Upon being released, he acted as if he were in pain. Believing him, Thomas turned his back again, and Vivian seized the opportunity to sucker punch Thomas in the same place that he had been hit with the rock. Thomas instantly cried out in pain, and fell to the ground. Vivian quickly jumped on top of Thomas, choking him. Thomas' friends tried to come to his rescue; however, they were strongly outnumbered by Vivian's acquaintances, and were quickly put in submissive holds themselves.

"This fight is between Thomas and me mate, Vivian." Henry told Charles as he held him in a headlock. Seeing Thomas helplessly holding his stomach in agony, Vivian laughed and picked up a boulder. All eyes were now intently focused on Vivian and Thomas.

Emily, who was being held by Stanley, screamed, "NOOO!" while Vivian lifted the boulder over his head with both hands. In agonizing pain, Thomas looked up at Vivian with fear in his eye. He knew that unless he was stopped, Vivian was only moments away from caving in his skull with the boulder, thus ending his life. Suddenly, from up a hill in the distance came the sound of furious growling and barking, sounds which echoed throughout the forest and could be heard for miles around. All eyes looked intently up that hill. What they vaguely saw was a creature with a huge head and big chest, foaming at the mouth. Behind this creature, they could see the setting sun, which that day was an unusually bright red; it almost looked like the sun and sky were bleeding. As all stared towards the creature, a voice in the crowd shouted, "Behold, the Hound of Hell!" At these words, the frightened crowd fled without getting a good look at the creature standing on the hill. They had all heard stories about the Hounds of Hell and were unwilling to risk their lives to find out if this was one of them. Vivian, along with his acquaintances, remained staring in awe. Thomas took advantage of Vivian's stare. Holding one hand on his stomach due to his pain, Thomas rolled so as to avoid being in a vulnerable position that would allow Vivian to cave in his skull. At this moment, Henry had one hand on Charles' throat, and the other hand cocked back in a fist. Henry would have pounded Charles in the face, had the creature standing on the hill showed up a second later.

Henry stared in fearful disbelief as he addressed Vivian. "I do not believe that is Angus up there." Vivian dropped his boulder but did not reply. He remained intrigued with the creature upon the hill.

However, Charles responded. "You are right Henry, for 'tis neither Vivian's dog up there, nor a hound of hell. Rather, 'tis Dare. Ye all should have been aware of that side of him! Because ye have troubled his master, all of your bloody lives may soon come to an end. I have heard those growls and barks once before. Shortly afterwards, his foe, the bull, was no more." Crouching on the top of the hill, Dare continued to growl. His massive fangs were fully exposed as he foamed at the mouth. He was eagerly waiting for Vivian or one of his acquaintances to move ever so slightly. Henry thought about what Charles had just said, then jumped to his feet, yelling and running for his life. Vivian followed, along with the rest of his acquaintances. Seeing this, Dare instantly charged down the hill at them in killing mode.

Thomas was very aware of this. He also knew that if Dare killed Vivian or any of his acquaintances, Dare would be killed himself. Therefore, he quickly rose to his feet, ignoring his pain and condition. When Dare approached, Thomas stood in his way, screaming despite his pain. "Halt! Do not attack!"

Dare slowed down. He growled and barked. His whole body shook as he stared deep into his master's eyes, telling him telepathically, "Please master, do not forbid me to tear Vivian apart! The thought of seeing him trying to kill you is too unbearable. I know you are concerned about me, but when it comes to your life, mine is irrelevant." After that thought, Dare snarled and barked as if to say, "Step aside master; do not deprive me of attacking your foe!"

Knowing that Dare was using every fiber of his being to obey him instead of chasing Vivian, Thomas pounced on his dog and wrapped his arms around him tightly as he said, "Control thyself; losing thy life over Vivian is not worth it. I know thy thoughts. Think though, what that would do to me, for how shall I live, having seen me best mate put to death?" Dare reluctantly submitted to his master. While in his master's grasp, he watched Vivian and his acquaintances run far away, up a big hill. His furious loud growls slowly turned into softer, quieter ones. A little while later, the growls stopped all together.

From the hill, at a long and safe distance, Vivian and his acquaintances stopped and looked at Thomas and his friends. Soon Angus appeared, stumbling slowly from over the hill where he had chased Dare. Angus ran much too hard. Desperately he gasped for air.

Henry was first to spot him. He pointed at him saying, "Look! There lies Angus!"

"Indeed!" Stanley replied, "And look, Dare has inflicted pain upon him!"

Dare watched Angus stumble from over the hill. He licked his master's face to acknowledge that he wasn't going to pursue Vivian any more today. He then broke free from his master's grasp and walked towards Angus with his head held down. Watching Dare approach Angus, Henry patted Vivian on the back, and said, "Sorry, matey, it looks like Dare is about to finish him off!" Vivian closed his eyes, clenched his fists, and pursed his lips as his head rolled backwards, not out of fear at the thought of his dog dying, but from humiliation, rage, and jealousy. Now everyone knew that he no longer had the best fighting dog of all the youth in town; and Vivian could not come to terms with the fact that Thomas now had the best fighting dog around.

Knowing that Angus was no match for or danger to his dog, Thomas yelled "Easy, Dare; do not harm him!" Dare came within one inch of Angus's face. Although exhausted, Angus tried to bite Dare's face off, but Dare's mongoose-like reflexes were much too fast for Angus. Dare jumped back, doing a three-sixty in a single leap. After this, he ran circles around Angus, while gently nipping at his tail and jumping over his back. The whole time, Angus desperately tried to bite Dare, but to no avail. After Dare played games with Angus for several minutes, Angus collapsed on the ground and laid there on his side, gasping for air. Angus now ignored Dare, who was nipping at him wanting to play some more. Angus was completely out of breath. He tried to get up, but couldn't. Dare soon turned around and walked back to his master and friends, who applauded the dog's performance, very proud that Dare had handled the situation without harming Angus, who was just following his corrupt master's orders to attack and kill. Thomas gave Dare lots of praise when he returned. "Good dog Dare! Good dog!" he said, while thumping on the dog's thick muscular chest. After that, Thomas and his friends walked away, all uninjured and with big smiles.

Henry again patted Vivian, who would have slugged Henry if it weren't for the fact that he could not beat him up. Vivian knew that Henry was about to make more sarcastic and derogatory comments. Therefore, he walked towards Angus with his back turned, brushing off Henry's hand as Henry told him, "Matey, you should feel grateful that Dare showed mercy in not tearing your dog apart, not to mention ourselves, as well."

Furious, Vivian turned back to Henry, and pointed his finger in Henry's face. "Never have I stated that my dog is faster than Dare, only that he is a better fighter. Angus could have, and would have, easily torn Dare apart, if not for Dare's cowardly running away for his bloody life!" Vivian turned back around and picked up his pace as he continued to walk towards Angus.

Hearing this, Henry chuckled as he sarcastically replied, "Aye, 'tis certain Dare looked mighty frightened, nipping at Angus while jumping back and forth over the top of him." Henry looked at his acquaintances, shaking his head while holding his index finger to his temple and making circular motions to indicate that Vivian was crazy. Stanley also said to Vivian sarcastically, "Fret not, matey; we all know your dog is a much better fighter than Dare. He probably would have proven it today by tearing Dare apart, if he had not been so tired." Vivian's acquaintances all continued to laugh at him.

Enraged, Vivian ground his teeth again and clenched his fists. He tried to ignore these comments while he walked over to Angus, who was still lying on his side on the ground, still trying to catch his breath. Vivian looked at him without compassion while shaking his head in disgust as he gave Angus a light kick in the stomach and whispered, "Get up, thou stupid dog. Thou hast embarrassed me today in front of all me mates." Angus soon rose to his feet. Panting very heavily, he sluggishly followed his master home.

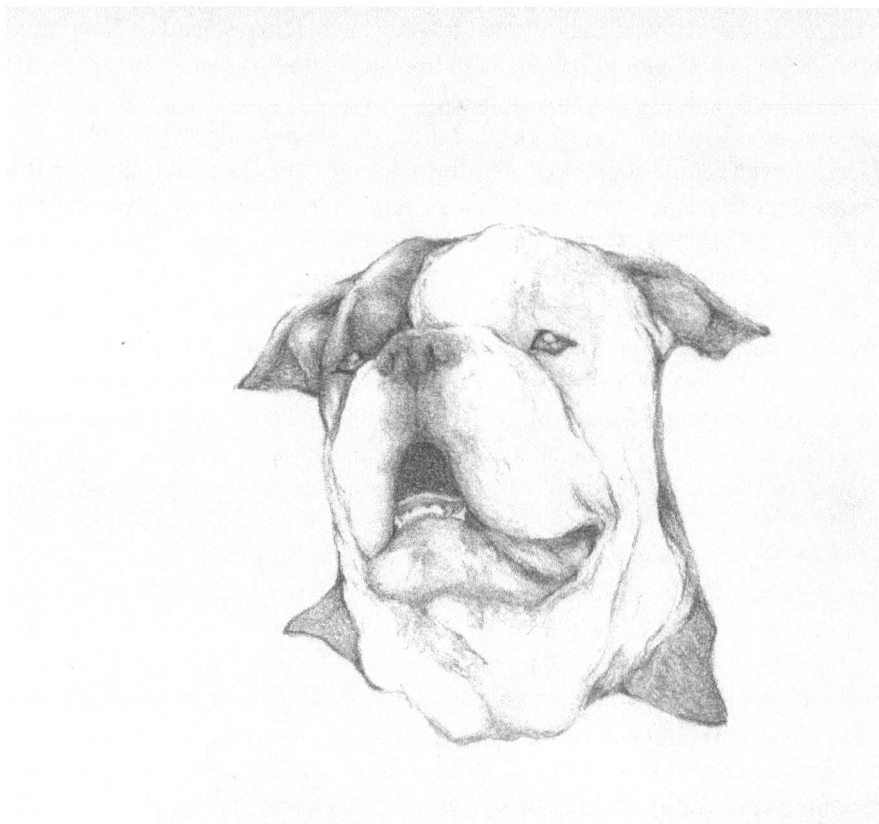

Dare's playful expression.

# CHAPTER XX
# THE ARROGANT, MOCKED

The next day, Vivian was still talking about how his dog would have torn Dare apart if Dare had not run away. Hearing this, all his acquaintances laughed.

"Hush now!" Vivian's acquaintance Jack, told him, annoyed. "Pray, do not take it as a personal insult that your dog is now a has-been, unlike Dare."

"Angus is no has-been!" Vivian replied with rage. "He is still the best bloody fighting dog around and shall prove all of you wrong!"

Rolling his eyes, Jack replied, "You are mad, Vivian, if you truly believe that.

Vivian's eyes opened wide as he proudly responded, "I do not merely believe; I do know that to be a fact, Jack! Before the sun sets, my fighting dog will prove that he is still the best in town."

Hearing this and seeing the look of pride and determination in Vivian's eyes, his acquaintances became troubled. They couldn't imagine that he was crazy enough to still believe that Angus had any chance of defeating Dare, especially after what they had witnessed yesterday.

Stammering and looking fearful, Stanley said, "That-is-fine Vivian, if you believe that. You had best make bloody sure that I am not around, though, if you do plan to put Dare to the test again!" The rest of Vivian's acquaintances said likewise.

Vivian thought, *"Oh no! All of you shall be there with me when Angus proves me right."* Vivian spoke confidently as he looked at Angus, who was lying on the ground while chewing the huge leg bone from a cow. "I have seen Angus tear apart the best fighting dogs in the pit! Never has he faced defeat! I do know that he will not disappoint me and will do the same to Dare!"

Henry glared at Vivian, while warning, "If you provoke Dare to fight while I am around, then after he has finished killing your dog, if he does not do likewise to you, I shall!"

Jack walked towards Angus, but when he came within seven feet of the dog, Angus turned and growled at him as if to say, "Come any closer to my cow bone and I will use one of your bones as a substitute for it."

Jack jumped back like a flash, saying, "Let us suppose that you are right, for the sake of argument, Vivian, and Angus is a better fighter than Dare. How can Angus prove you right, for he can not catch Dare?"

With his right hand to his chin, Vivian looked to the ground and thought, *"Jack has a good point. What can I do to make sure that Dare doesn't run away frightened again?"* At that moment, Vivian heard all his acquaintances whistling and making crude comments and facial expressions at Emily and Sara, who were on their way to Thomas' house and just happened to pass by. Vivian suddenly came up with an evil plan. His eyes opened wide, for he realized that if Thomas were to see Angus about to attack Emily, he would command Dare to defend her, instead of ordering his dog to run away. Vivian guessed that the girls were heading over to Thomas' house, so he ordered Angus to heel and come with him as he followed the girls. Vivian motioned to his acquaintances as he said, "Follow me lads; let us see where these beautiful young ladies are going! Perhaps they would like our company."

"Why yes indeed, sounds mighty good to me," Stanley replied, with big lustful smiles, they walked in back of the girls, following them closely.

Vivian, with Angus, walked closest to the girls. "Good day, young ladies. Methought ye could use our protection, so, being perfect gentlemen, we decided to follow ye to make sure that you arrive safely at your destination." As Vivian said this, his acquaintances mumbled disgusting kissing sounds and crude comments at the girls. The girls knew that these fellows were trouble and up to no good, so they picked up their pace.

Sara turned, glancing at Angus while she continued to walk quickly. "Our thanks for your offer, but we prefer to walk alone."

Vivian gave a sinister chuckle. "Ha! Now, that is not very polite. Us nice lads (and the dog) care about your safety, and insist on following you." Emily and Sara were frightened by hearing this, as well as all the whistling in back of them. They glanced quickly at one another, and then took off running towards Thomas' house.

Seeing the girls running, Angus's instinct was to chase and attack. Vivian knew this and quickly grabbed him by the neck to prevent him from chasing the girls. "Wait a minute!" Vivian ordered his dog. "Let us wait till they get closer to Thomas' home before thou dost attack." Angus growled loudly at the word *attack*. Vivian kept one hand on Angus's collar while they followed the girls. Half a mile later, when they were close to Thomas' house, Vivian let go of Angus's collar, pointed at Emily, and commanded, "Attack now!" Emily saw Vivian point and give the attack command. However, instead of running towards Thomas' house, she ran for her life towards the woods. Emily had never run so fast in her entire life. She hurdled over trees, bushes, and rocks. Angus was following behind her, and was foaming at the mouth.

Vivian followed, screaming, "No! No! Not out in the woods! Run towards Thomas' house!" His screams were to no avail. Emily and Angus kept running farther away from Thomas' house. All of Vivian's acquaintances froze in shock. They knew Vivian was a bad person, but never imagined he would stoop so low as to have Angus kill a helpless girl.

Henry shouted furiously, "Vivian, you bloody stupid fool! Call Angus off! If he harms Emily, we shall all be in tremendous trouble." Vivian responded by commanding Angus to stop, but his commands were to no avail, for Angus was now in full-fledged attack mode, and was focused solely on Emily. Angus quickly closed the gap between himself and Emily. At this time, Thomas and Dare were out playing fetch the stick. At the moment Emily screamed in fear, Dare was in midair, about to catch the stick. Hearing Emily scream, Dare completely ignored the stick and ran faster than the wind towards the sound, followed by a cloud of dust from his feet. Witnessing this, Thomas whistled in disbelief; he had never seen anything move faster. Unlike Dare, Thomas didn't hear any screams, but he knew that something was definitely wrong. It was not like Dare to ignore a stick thrown for him, especially in midair. Thomas followed, chasing the cloud of dust left by Dare. Angus was just about caught up with Emily who was running, moving side-to-side and jumping over trees that had fallen. Angus' mouth was wide open, and he was trying to take a big chunk out of her. He soon got a big piece of Emily's dress, and ripped it almost completely off. Emily staggered and put one hand on the ground to help keep her balance, soon regaining her composure. She continued running, without looking back. Emily attempted to hurdle over another tree, but her right foot scraped against a small branch, causing her to fly in the air and land flat on her face; this also caused a bloody nose and lip, and a scraped left arm from the fall. Helplessly, she remained on the ground, more than half naked from Angus having ripped her dress. Too frightened to look up for fear she would see Angus flying at her, Emily kept her face near the ground as she cried out, "God! Help me!" At that moment, about to attack with his jaws wide open, Angus was in the air, hurdling over the same tree in which Emily had tried to hurdle over. From the opposite direction of the approaching Angus, Emily felt a tail smack her in the back of her head. It was Dare, and his timing was impeccable. He met Angus head on in midair, and wrapped his jaws around Angus's throat. The force of momentum from Dare's jump, combined with his powerful neck muscles, enabled him to bash Angus headfirst into the ground, scattering dirt and grass everywhere. Angus was knocked completely unconscious. Dare concerned Emily might have been attacked by Angus and badly injured switched his attention to her. He looked and sniffed at Emily to make sure she was all right, as Emily lay shaking with fear. She thought Angus was the one sniffing and lurking over her, about to attack. Her face remained close to the ground, and she did not look up. Dare did not smell any of Angus's saliva on Emily, nor did he see any bite marks on her, and he could see from the movements that she made as she shook that her bones were not broken, so Dare knew that Emily was only frightened, not badly injured. Dare then turned, and with his head low to the ground, looked at Vivian and all of Vivian's acquaintances. Once again, his massive, razor-sharp fangs were fully exposed as he foamed at the mouth. Vivian and his acquaintances were shaking far worse than was Emily. After witnessing what Dare had just done, they looked at him in disbelief, as if they were looking at the grim reaper himself. None of them said a word, but all turned and ran for their lives with shear terror. Dare chased Vivian and was just about to catch him, when at the last moment, Vivian very intelligently jumped up and grabbed a tree branch and quickly climbed up the tree, while Dare jumped at him, snapping his jaws a few inches away. Together, Henry and Stanley climbed another tree next to the tree Vivian had climbed.

Emily slowly stopped shaking. "Wait a minute," she said to herself, "How was it possible for Angus's tail to hit me in the front of my head when he was coming at me from the other direction?" Immediately after saying this, Emily heard Dare bark from a distance. "Dare must have saved me, just as he saved Thomas!" Emily said, putting the pieces together. She opened up her eyes and was momentarily terrified. She screamed, "AAHH!" because the first thing she saw was Angus lying right next to her. Seeing that Angus didn't respond or move, she realized that Angus was either dead or unconscious, but in any case, was in no state to harm her. Emily then rose to her feet and walked over to Dare, who at the moment was furiously trying to climb the tree that Vivian was perched in, and tear him apart.

Henry looked at Dare with great fear. He soon figured out that Vivian's evil plan was to command Angus to attack Emily so as to make Dare fighting mad, preventing him from turning and running as he had the last time. Henry ripped a small branch off of his tree and threw it at Vivian. "Damn you, Vivian!" Henry shouted, "You are a fool! Did I not tell you that if you tested Dare again, I did not want to be around? Your foolish act has now put our lives in great danger, along with your own pathetic life!"

Vivian took deep breaths in an attempt to gather his nerves. This wasn't easy. Not only did he have Dare attempting to bite his face off, but now he had to dodge tree branches that were being thrown at him by Henry and Stanley. Vivian soon realized that Dare was not capable of climbing up to his perch in the tree. He looked over at Henry and Stanley and told them, "Oh, do just calm yourselves, ye two buffoons. None of our lives is in danger from this stupid dog. Look at him! There is no way that he can climb these trees and attack us up here. Do be patient; help will soon come to us."

As both Stanley and Henry continued to break branches from their tree and throw them at Vivian, the frightened Stanley replied, "Do not say another word about Dare! 'Tis you who are the buffoon! I do begin to seriously believe that this is not just a dog, but the leader of the Hounds of Hell, the dogs we have all heard nightmarish stories about, and now, thanks to you, Dare's about to send us to hell.

Vivian looked at Henry and Stanley with disbelief. "And you call me a fool? Stanley, what you have just said is proof that you are the fool!" Upon saying *fool*, Vivian was hit in the head with a branch thrown by Stanley. "Ouch! Stop throwing branches at me, the two of ye." Vivian said, while feeling his head and dodging more branches.

Realizing that he wasn't getting anywhere by jumping up and down and barking at Vivian, Dare began to bite the base of Vivian's tree. He quickly ripped out big chunks of bark.

Seeing this, all three lads trembled with fear, especially Vivian. Stanley slapped his forehead saying, "You simply do not know when to shut your bloody mouth, do you Vivian? You and your dog deserve to die, which, by the looks of the way Dare is attacking your tree, is going to happen soon. Henry and I, on the other hand, do not deserve to die."

Henry pleaded with Dare in a terrified tone of voice. "Dare, pray have mercy on Stanley and me for being with this bloody fool. We honestly tried to tell him not to bother you and your friends. Unfortunately, he just wouldn't listen to us. So, we plead for your wrath to be bestowed upon Vivian alone!"

Vivian, seeing his tree only a few more chomps away from falling to the ground, started to panic. "Oh my God! I am going to die!" Vivian exclaimed, as his tree began to sway. At this moment, Thomas showed up. He bent over from the waist, with his hands on his legs, trying to catch his breath that he had lost from running. Seeing Thomas, Vivian sighed with relief, and said, "Thank goodness you are here. Your mad beast is trying to kill me. Call him off at once!"

When he raised his head, the first thing Thomas saw was Emily, more than half naked with a torn dress, and bleeding from her face and left arm. Thomas assumed that Vivian and his acquaintances had raped her. For the first time in his life, Thomas was overtaken by rage. Running towards Vivian's tree, he screamed like a madman. "AHH! AHH!" Thomas, roaring, commanded Dare to "Leave at once!" as he pushed him away as hard as he could. When Dare backed up, Thomas wrapped his arms around the tree in which Vivian was perched, and shook it as hard as he could, causing the tree, along with Vivian, to fall to the ground. Vivian staggered to his feet. Upon rising, Vivian was quickly tackled and brought to the ground again by Thomas. Once Vivian was pinned, Thomas began punching Vivian in the face, causing blood to quickly gush everywhere. When Vivian was nearly unconscious, Thomas jumped to his feet, kicking Vivian in the ribs and shouting as he bruised them, "You have just hurt me and me matey's for the last time, for you are now about to die!" Bleeding all over the place, Vivian tried to rise to his feet. In doing so, he was greeted by a foot in the face, courtesy of Thomas. This caused Vivian to flip over backwards, and knocked him out cold.

Henry and Stanley began to plead with Thomas as he was beating the bloody crap out of Vivian. "Stop, Thomas! We do plead, have mercy! You are killing him!" Thomas didn't pay any attention to them, for he was solely focused on attacking Vivian.

Knowing that one more blow would probably kill Vivian, if he weren't already dead, Emily wrapped her arms around Thomas and cried, "Pray, no more!"

Feeling Emily's breasts and heavenly body half naked snuggled close to his own, Thomas became even more enraged, for he thought, *"That bloody piece of trash has just violated the lady of my dreams, stealing her virginity, which I was hoping would be reserved for me one day."* Out of rage, Thomas moved Emily's arms off of him and pushed her aside, causing Emily to trip on a rock. "I am sorry Emily; but there is no way that anybody, not even thyself, can prevent me from killing this bloody bastard for what he did to thee."

Emily cried all the more, "No, do not, I beg of thee." Thomas ignored Emily's plea and focused completely on his goal of using his right leg to cave in Vivian's head, who was still lying helpless on the ground.

Henry and Stanley both screamed, "Have mercy!" as Emily cried. She remained on the ground, shaking her head and staring while Thomas approached Vivian as if in slow motion. Emily knew that there was nothing she could say or do now to stop Thomas from killing Vivian. With his right leg fully extended behind him Thomas started to swing his leg at Vivian's head with every fiber in his being, intending to kick it like a field goal kicker tries to kick a sixty-yard field goal. At the last fraction of a second, Dare grabbed Thomas from the back by his collar and threw him to the ground, just as Thomas' foot scraped against Vivian's hair. With his paws on Thomas' shoulders, Dare kept Thomas pinned there. Thomas tried to get free from his dog, but soon realized that he was not strong enough to break his beloved dogs hold on him. Thomas lay on the ground crying like a baby, as Dare licked his tears. Thomas thought Emily had been raped and would never again be the same, and also thought that he would now probably hang, for he thought he had just killed Vivian.

By now, a long time had passed. Henry and Stanley were still up in the tree, and were looking down, annoyed. Dare kept his master pinned to the ground, thinking that his master would try to finish Vivian off if he were released. Thomas kept asking Emily repeatedly whether she had been violated, while Emily sat next to Thomas, telling him over and over that she was fine and had not in fact been raped. Thomas didn't believe her, so questioned her again and again.

Emily shook her head in disgust. She bent over and looked down at Thomas as she started yelling at him. "I am becoming rather tired of constantly telling thee that bloody scum did not violate me, nor did any of his bloody friends!"

Henry and Stanley nodded their heads in agreement. "The lady is telling the truth." Henry added, "We will swear on the Holy Bible. Now pray, call off your dog, we humbly beg, so we can come down out of this tree." Thomas and Emily ignored them. Every now and then, Henry tried to come down from the tree, but when he did so, Dare turned towards him with his huge fangs exposed. Seeing this, Henry hastily climbed back up to the top of the tree, trembling with fear.

Emily finally had had enough. She was tired of going around in circles, trying to convince Thomas she hadn't been raped. She rolled her eyes, and took a deep breath as she said, "Unfortunately, there is but one way to prove that I am telling the truth when I say that I was not violated. Do thou remember, Thomas, that I take no pleasure in proving that to thee in this degrading manner. I will probably never forgive thee, either, for making me do what I am about to do!" Emily patted Dare on the neck. "Good dog! Thou mayest release him now; thy master will no longer be violent." Dare had faith in her and got off of his master as Emily stood directly over Thomas' face. She pulled her panties down, while taking Thomas' hand and placing it on her vagina. Thomas' hand shook as if he were having a seizure, and his eyes looked like they were about to pop out of their sockets. His mouth opened wide, as he babbled like an idiot, but no words come out. Emily's vagina was dry and not abused. Thomas now knew without a shadow of a doubt that Emily was telling the truth when she said that she had not been violated. Henry and Stanley stared with wide eyes as they tried to get a good look at Emily's private parts from the tree. Both stretched out their necks, which caused both of them to lose their grips on the tree and come crashing to the ground at the same time.

Once Emily was convinced that Thomas believed her, she glared at him angrily and slapped his face. "I do surely hope thou art satisfied, Thomas Avery Gentry," Emily told him as she pulled up her panties. Thomas remained lying on the ground, babbling like an idiot.

Dare turned and looked at Henry and Stanley who were lying on the ground, holding their backs and legs, and moaning in pain. Dare walked towards them, growling, with his head low to the ground. Their pain was quickly forgotten. Henry urinated in his pants while looking at Dare as he begged Thomas, "Pray, call your dog off. Let us live, for we have done harm to no one."

Stanley nodded his head in agreement, pleading, "We promise that we shall never again harm you, nor any of your friends."

Coming out of his trance, Thomas told them, "Keep quiet and do not move." Thomas slowly rose to his feet, and then put both hands on the back of his head. Looking over at Vivian, he said, "I have just killed him; surely I shall hang." Thomas covered his eyes, feeling great remorse, not so much because he thought he had just killed someone, but mainly because he had never dreamed how good Emily's vagina would feel, and now he was afraid that he was never going to ever feel it again. Thomas fell to the ground on his knees, looking down and shaking his head back and forth, while hyperventilating. Dare walked over to his master and licked his face, knowing he was in great distress. Thomas gave Dare a bear hug, kissing his cheek. "I am going to really miss thee, mate."

Dare knew that his master thought that he had killed Vivian and feared that he would be in enormous trouble for it, so Dare slapped his master across the face with his right paw, as if to say, "Do not worry master. Dry those pathetic tears. Haven't I proven that I will always protect you?" Dare walked over to Vivian, lifted his hind leg, and took the biggest piss of his entire life right on Vivian's face, causing Vivian to wake up as Dare's urine gushed into his face, mouth and eyes. Seeing and tasting urine, Vivian vomited a large amount of it, and then rubbed his eyes and shook some of the urine out of his hair in total disgust. Seeing Vivian alive, Thomas' first thoughts were, *"Yes I am going to live. Maybe I will have the extremely great pleasure of feeling Emily's private parts again some day."* Thomas hugged and kissed Dare over and over saying, "Good dog, Dare! Good dog!"

Everybody looked at Thomas as if he was demented, believing that Thomas was praising Dare for having urinated in Vivian's face. Disgusted, Emily shook her head at Thomas. "Hast thou gone mad," she scolded, "praising thy dog for urinating in someone's face? Thou hast just revealed an evil and demented aspect which I do not like."

"Heavens, no!" Thomas explained, "My praise to Dare was for waking Vivian up, for I believed that Vivian was dead, and that I would surely hang."

Hearing this, Charles gave a quick chuckle as he defended his friend. "You have to admit, Emily, that Vivian deserved that, and it was rather hilarious."

Emily didn't respond with words, although the little smirk on her face said, "I do agree Charles."

Thomas, thinking about what had just happened, glanced at Emily, looking at her from head to toe with lust in his eyes and admiring her beauty. Being the perfect gentleman, Thomas took off his shirt to wrap around Emily's waist to help cover up her nakedness. Then Thomas took Emily's left hand, got down on one knee and begged for forgiveness for not believing her.

Emily pulled her hand quickly away. She narrowed her eyes at him as she crossed her arms. "Thou dost realize, Thomas Avery Gentry, that I did not wish to prove what I was telling thee in that degrading way."

"Yes, I do, my lady." Thomas acknowledged, "I am truly sorry that I influenced thee to do what thou didst," But he was thinking, *"I am not so sure that I really mean that."*

Emily slapped Thomas across his face again, saying. "I am still really upset with thee, Thomas Gentry."

Thomas took Emily's hand again, closed his eyes, bowed his head and kissed Emily's hand. "I know my lady, and rightfully so. I humbly beg thee, my lady, to give me a chance to make it up." Emily looked at Thomas as he bowed with a touch of lust for him herself. She noticed that the muscles of his bare back and chest were extremely attractive. Emily could tell by the way Thomas was acting that he was in love with her. She thought, *"I hope, someday soon, Thomas will ask for my hand in marriage, in which case I will have the chance to act on my carnal desires."* Emily snapped herself out of her trance as she smacked Thomas on the back of his head with her right hand, saying "Rise up! Thou art making a fool of thyself! I will consider forgiving thee, as long as thou dost never speak of what happened to anyone!"

With a sigh of relief, Thomas rose to his feet. "So be it, my lady. I shall be a gentleman, and will keep my mouth shut." Thomas turned as he gave Henry and Stanley the evil eye: "Ye two shall also remain silent, lest a fate be bestowed upon ye worse than what almost happened to your matey."

Henry and Stanley shook with fear at the thought, and Henry replied, "Do not fret, young master; we both swear that we shall not say a word." Stanley nervously nodded his head in agreement.

At that moment, Angus gained consciousness and slowly rose to his feet, his head covered with dirt and grass. In a daze, Angus staggered over to Vivian, who sat up, also in a daze. Thomas told Stanley and Henry, "Ye two are free to leave now. Mark my words, I will hold ye both to your vows."

Happy to finally be able to leave, Henry replied, nodding his head with a smile, "Our thanks, Master Thomas. We shall keep our vows." After this acknowledgement, Henry and Stanley immediately started to walk away.

Thomas was shocked to see this, for they were going to leave without Vivian and Angus, so he shouted at them. "Wait! Wait!"

Cringing, the two stopped as Stanley responded, "Yes, Master Thomas." Both were thinking, *"Oh no, what now?"*

Thomas pointed at Vivian and Angus, "Are you not going to help them home?"

Stanley looked at Vivian who smelled of urine and was still wet from it. Stanley and Henry both knew that Vivian was in no shape to walk home by himself, and needed an arm around him in order to walk. But they also knew that whoever put his arm around Vivian would become wet with Dare's urine.

Giving himself a quick slap in the head, Stanley answered Thomas, "I do not know what we were thinking. Certainly we shall help them home," then he patted Henry on the shoulder, saying, "Me matey Henry shall help Vivian as I do likewise to Angus."

Henry shook his head, sweeping Vivian's arm off his shoulder. "Oh no! You help Vivian and I shall help Angus!"

As the two argued, Vivian was lying on the ground. As he spit out blood, he addressed Thomas, saying, "Your dog may be a better fighter than Angus, but my uncle Lord Riley's dog Terror could tear him apart and chew him up into little pieces." Hearing this, Henry and Stanley stopped arguing, and focused their undivided attention on Vivian, for they knew these two powerful and agile creatures had the same blood flowing through their veins. If there ever were a fight between these two canine brothers, it would probably be the bloodiest dogfight in history.

Filled with even more rage at hearing this, Thomas stood directly in front of Vivian, stared deep into his eyes, and in a furious tone of voice, said "I must hear you swear to God and vow with your life that you shall never again try to hurt any of me mates or force my dog to fight." Vivian did not want to make any vows, especially with God involved, for he knew if he had Terror by his side, or perhaps someday another dog that had a chance against Dare, he would put that dog to the test. So Vivian tried to ignore Thomas, by looking away and hoping that Thomas wouldn't push the issue. However, Thomas did push the issue; he moved even closer to Vivian, screaming in rage as he kicked dirt in Vivian's face, "Acknowledge me! Acknowledge me now! Or before the sun sets, your blood will be spilled all over the ground! Let me now hear your vow!"

The dirt going into Vivian's face and lungs made him cough, and he spit out blood while holding his painfully bruised ribs. Looking up at Thomas, Vivian saw eyes like fire. He thought, *"Thomas surely looks as if he is going to add force to what he just said."* Without hesitation, Vivian raised both hands in surrender, saying, "Alright! Alight! I do now swear to God and do vow with my life that I shall never try to hurt any of your family members or mates ever again. Are you pleased now?"

Thomas continued to stare at Vivian with eyes like a raging fires, as he answered,"No, I am not pleased. This shall be the last time that I grant mercy and allow you to live. Do always remember that if you break your vow, you shall not have only my wrath to fear, but the wrath of the Almighty." After warning Vivian, Thomas turned and patted Dare on the head, then the two walked away with Emily. Thomas tried to hold Emily's hand, but she pulled her hand away and crossed her arms, acting as though she were still mad at him, which she wasn't. Emily was just playing games as Thomas and Dare walked her safely home.

After Thomas and his friends had left, Henry and Stanley were still arguing about which one of them would put his arm around Vivian and help him walk home.

# CHAPTER XXI
# CHALLENGE TO THE DEATH

As stories continued to spread about Dare killing Bulldread, the popularity of bull-bating spread like wildfire. People would come to Lord Riley's tents from miles around to watch five dogs released one at a time to attack a large bull. The first four dogs were almost certain to die, but by the fifth dog, the bull sometimes started to unwind and was soon to die. People paid a pretty penny to watch. At these events, large wagers were always placed. People who attended these events always watched in awe as they witnessed fearless dogs being tossed more than twenty feet in the air, and fighting to the death. People began to ponder the question of whether a dog could actually kill a huge bull without any help from any of the other dogs, as described in the stories that were being spread.

One day, Lord Edward Lewis, one of England's richest lords, who was a devout fan of bull baiting and owner of several powerful bulls, propositioned Lord Riley in hopes of finding out. "Lord Riley, my comrades and I would be willing to pay a good deal money if you could produce a dog worthy of fighting a bull by himself. Can this be arranged?"

With a smile, Lord Riley answered loudly, "'Tis true? Are ye all willing to pay a good deal?"

"Yes."

"Indeed," answered the people around them, with bloodthirsty eyes.

With greed gleaming in his eyes, Lord Riley responded, "Fellow comrades, such a fight shall be arranged. Terror, the best fighting dog of all time, brother to the dog who killed Bulldread, shall likewise attempt a fight to the death." Hearing this, the people were in awe and in great anticipation. Lord Edward responded in a challenging tone, "Will Terror likewise fight a bull survivor of the pit, such as Brahma The Bull, or me own Enormous Elias, as you claim his brother Dare did? Or shall he be sheltered against an unproven, unworthy opponent?"

"Terror shall fight the bull which shall make me the most mon- (Lord Riley stopped himself from saying money.) I mean that you most desire." The people in the crowd gasped and rolled their eyes, knowing that Lord Riley only cared about money, not about what they desired.

Lord Edward answered, "Without a doubt, that would be Enormous Elias." The crowd all agreed with Lord Edward.

"Are you sure? For what chance would Terror hold? Enormous Elias is a seven time survivor of the pit, the killer of several of my best dogs!"

"Yes, Enormous Elias," echoed the crowd.

Lord Edward added, "You claim that Terror is the best fighting dog of all time. You can prove it beyond a shadow of a doubt with a victory over Elias."

Lord Riley pondered the situation as the crowd eagerly anticipated his answer. "So it shall be." Lord Riley knew better than anyone Terror's exceptional fighting ability and inner rage. He had downplayed Terror so the odds would heavily favor Elias. Lord Riley was going to bet all money made on this fight and then some on Terror.

"When will this fight take place?" asked Lord Edward.

"Prepare Elias. For it shall be soon."

Lord Riley started to walk away as the crowd pursued with intense curiosity.

"When?"

"When?"

"When shall it be?"

Lord Riley smiled before turning around, knowing that the crowd was under his thumb. "I shall announce the date of the fight when Terror is trained well enough for all to receive their money's worth." The crowd sighed and looked annoyed, unhappy that no date had been given.

"Heed me words, for what ye see shall surely be the best damn bloodiest fight in history." Lord Riley stirred people's curiosity even more as he left them with these words and an even bigger greedy smile, knowing that after this fight, he could be the richest lord of all.

Lord Edward addressed his comrades. "Lord Riley is a fool if he believes that his dog hath any chance of defeating Elias."

"How much will you wager on your bull to win?" asked a comrade.

"I shall bet half of my riches!"

"Wooo!" They all responded, for they knew the size of Lord Edward's fortune.

"Why so surprised? I have no doubts that my bull shall win. If five of Lord Riley's dogs cannot defeat Elias, what chance would one dog have?"

Over the next several weeks, Lord Riley focused all his attention on Terror's training. He built Terror's muscles up even more by having him pull a horse carriage for several miles every other day, gradually adding heavy metal to the carriage. Soon, Terror was able to pull over fifty times his body weight. Terror was a natural at pulling and needed no assistance. Ignorant of this fact, Lord Riley whipped him, thinking that this would make him pull harder. This affected Terror by making him even angrier, and made him want to kill everything in sight. He became so vicious that

Terror was forbidden to have any contact with humans or livestock when Lord Riley wasn't around. Most of his time was spent imprisoned in a small filthy cage. Lord Riley even had to pay close attention when breeding Terror because immediately after breeding, Terror would attack his mate. When he wasn't pulling, Terror's days off consisted of sprinting and fighting cattle. They started him off on small cattle. Terror instinctively locked his jaws on the cow's nose, similar to the way Dare had locked his jaws on Bulldread. Gradually, Lord Riley used bigger cattle. Soon Terror was able to take on medium sized bulls. Lord Riley, not wishing to risk any serious injuries and losing the biggest pay day of his life, always had four other fighting dogs on hand in case Terror looked like he might need help. On one occasion, it appeared that Terror was having a difficult time contending with an average sized bull. Without hesitation, Lord Riley sent the four additional dogs to Terror's aid. Terror became enraged when, out of the corner of his eye, he saw the other dogs approaching. This gave him the extra strength needed to slam the bull face first in the dirt, as the dogs neared. Immediately afterward, Terror attacked Chad, the biggest of the four dogs, and by the throat, brought Chad to the ground. With a demonic grin, Lord Riley whipped Terror on the back, commanding, "Release,"

With a growl, Terror released Chad, standing over him with the thought, *"One more second and I would have crushed your throat!"* Chad ran far away from Terror, and the three other dogs did the same.

Well-pleased, Lord Riley responded with a twisted smile, "Terror, thou art the fiercest, most heartless beast, for not only dost thou now show no mercy to any foe, but thou also dost show no mercy to those desiring to help!" Lord Riley paused, giving a quick whip near Terror's ear. Terror growled, but avoided eye contact, knowing that his master would consider eye contact a challenge and would whip him thoroughly. "I have trained and whipped thee well." (Lord Riley always took full credit for his dogs' fighting ability.) "Now thou art ready to face Elias." Switching his attention to Chad, Lord Riley whipped him, saying, "Had I had six other dogs with half of Terror's fighting ability, I would have let him crush thy throat!"

Confident that Terror was now a worthy adversary for Enormous Elias, Lord Riley announced the date and time of this fight to the death. Never before had a dog, fighting alone, taken on a bull, in public. Lord Riley knew that this spectacle was going to be bloody, just like the one he had witnessed with Dare. There was a good chance that Terror would not come out of this fight alive, and even if he did, there was no way that he would come through it without injuries. Therefore, before the fight, Lord Riley bred Terror with an awful lot of females because he thought, *"After this fight, Terror will probably never be able to breed again, so, I had better milk my best fighting dog for all he is worth."* Lord Riley set the date of the fight for a Sunday morning, only five weeks before Christmas. Lord Riley always held his bull baiting events on Sunday mornings. This angered a lot of people who attended church, but Lord Riley didn't care. When questioned about the day and time, he would say, "Go to church, then. I am not preventing you or anyone from attending church. If you would rather go to church than miss me bloody Sunday extravaganza, go ahead!"

Priests pleaded with Lord Riley. "Pray, Lord Riley, change the day and time. It will not affect the outcome of your attendance. Whenever you hold an event, church attendance is down by at least fifty percent."

Pleased to hear this, Lord Riley would respond, "Sunday is the day I choose. If that causes a problem for you, then change the day and time of the church service!" A few members of the clergy preached against not forsaking the Sabbath and against the evil that they felt bull bating to be. By the following Sunday, attendance at those churches had dropped by about fifty percent.

The churches knew that they couldn't compete with bull baiting. Priests stopped talking to their congregations about how wrong or evil they felt bull bating was, for fear half their congregation would leave to join a church that didn't preach against their favorite sport.

One priest, Father Van Dirk, approached Lord Riley one day when they were alone asking, "Why do you hold bull baiting events on the Sabbath? Why not on a different day?" Lord Riley answered with a sinister smile. "Because 'tis the highest form of flattery to me, seeing so called God-fearing people break the Sabbath in order to attend me bloody spectacle."

Father Van Dirk, baffled by Lord Riley's response, pointed at him with a raised voice. "Doest thou not fear God? Hearken, thou shall be held accountable for the brothers and sisters forsaking the Sabbath to attend thy spectacle!"

Hearing this, Lord Riley laughed in Father Van Dirk's face. "Do not preach to me, Father Dirk! I do not belong to your church. If you want to preach, go to church and preach!"

Father Van Dirk, angry, held his bible up high. "Heed these words, heathen! Someday almighty God shall pour out his wrath upon you, unless repentance comes from thy evil ways!"

"Worry not, jealous Father!" Lord Riley replied laughing even louder. "I have news to convey to you. There is no God! You and your congregation are all bloody fools! Half of your congregation would rather worship my dogs than worship God!"

This made Father Van Dirk lean back in shock as he crossed himself. "You have been warned! Unless repentance comes, the wrath of the Almighty shall be bestowed upon you! The Angel of Death's sting shall be without mercy!"

Lord Riley laughed even louder. Taking out a large pouch full of money, he held it up to Father Van Dirk mockingly. "Do you see this, Van Dirk? This is my God! If your so called Angel of Death comes for me, I shall buy my way free!"

As Lord Riley turned and started to walk away, Father Van Dirk yelled, "What shall it profit a man if he gains the whole world and loses his immortal soul?"

Lord Riley responded, "Hah! Right!" as he kept walking, shaking his head with a perturbed wave of his hand.

Word that Terror would fight against Elias spread over England faster than gangrene. Even Queen Mary had arranged to attend this bloody event. Charles saw a handbill advertising the event on a wall. When nobody was looking, he took it down and brought it to Thomas. Seeing the handbill, Thomas was greatly disturbed. It read, "Come witness the Legendary Bulldog, Terror, the best fighting, fiercest dog in history, contend against Enormous Elias, one of the few bull survivors of the pit, killer of five bulldogs at once, in a fight that shall indeed be a blood bath to the death." A picture on the handbill depicted Terror biting Enormous Elias on the nose, hanging on, while blood spurted all over. The image of Terror in the picture looked identical to his brother Dare when he killed Bulldread.

Seeing this picture, Thomas closed his eyes, remembering how Dare almost died. Then he opened his eyes, and crumpled up the handbill, throwing it down and swearing, "Damn that Lord Riley!" Thomas expressed his rage: "As long as I shall live, I shall never attend any of his bloody spectacles!" Charles reluctantly commented with his head hung low, "It may be wrong; however, I am rather curious to see if Dare's brother fights and defeats Elias in the same manner that Dare defeated Bulldread."

With raging eyes, Thomas stared into Charles's eyes, scolding, "I am most appalled at thee, Charles, for even considering attending such a bloody spectacle. Wasn't it bad enough to see a dog fight a bull once when I was attacked?"

"Thou art right," Charles responded, knowing his friend's strong convictions towards bull bating. "I do not know what I was thinking. That thought must have been of the devil."

Thomas shook his head in utter disgust at the thought. *"Every day, I pray for the outlaw of bull bating, but unfortunately, the bloody sport keeps growing more and more popular. This disturbs me."*

Charles nodded his head in agreement. "I shall also pray for bull bating to be outlawed, especially on the Sabbath."

Hearing Charles's change of heart, Thomas calmed down. Patting Charles on the shoulder, he replied, "We need to also pray for the people who attend these spectacles. They would rather see a bloody Sabbath than attend church. These people are throwing away God's protecting shield, allowing themselves to be easier targets for the Devil."

Charles quickly nodded his head in agreement, but at the same time thought, *"Thomas, sometimes thou canst be so fanatical!"*

Thomas turned to his dog, and patted him on the head. "It breaks my heart to hear that thy brother is soon to fight a bull for people's sick amusement. I do surely wish that thy brother had been with thee when thou wert found. He would be a loving, happy dog like thee, with his tail wagging all the time, too."

After Thomas had said this to Dare, he held his head down near Dare's face, with eyes closed. Hugging Dare's big thick neck, he shed a tear, whispering, "What if Lord Riley had kept thee? And thou wert treated like thy brother?" This was a very disturbing thought.

Charles, noticing the pure love in Dare's eyes, commented, "Except when someone crosses thy path, I have never in my life seen a nicer creature than thy dog. It is hard to believe that he has a brother half as mean as Terror."

"I agree. Terror's wicked master, Lord Riley, must have really been abusive."

A little while later, Thomas rose to his feet, acting as if he was all right, but his heart was in agony about news of the upcoming spectacle. He told Charles, "I would like to be alone now with me dog." The two turned and walked away. Charles watched them leave and could tell that Thomas was distressed by the way he held his head, low and swaying.

A couple of weeks later, on the night before Lord Riley's spectacle, Thomas had a strange nightmare. He dreamed that he was at the fight, in the front row close to the center of the arena. He didn't see the fight because he was looking the other way, toward the bloodthirsty crowd. In his dream, he saw several bloodthirsty people yelling and cheering, encouraging the bull to kill Dare's brother. Suddenly, Thomas saw a giant man in the very back, dressed in white and standing about ten feet tall. When Thomas saw the giant, he no longer heard the roaring crowd. The giant was holding Dare, as a puppy, in his right hand and Terror, as a puppy, in his left. The puppies were held close to each other. Thomas watched the puppies happily play at fighting, while wiggling their little tails. Suddenly, both puppies stopped playing and looked at Thomas, troubled. They began begging for his help in human voices as they began to bleed. The puppies soon disappeared, first Dare, and then Terror.

With blood dripping from both of his hands, the giant spoke to Thomas. "Thomas, Thomas, you must promise to attend this event. You soon shall awaken with a bad stomachache. Thomas, Thomas, you must attend this event." After the giant said this, Thomas screamed in his dream. "I shall, I promise." Thomas saw a huge, bright white light, moments before waking up. Sweating, and with a very bad stomachache, Thomas forced himself to his feet, then rolled backwards onto his bed as he told his parents, "I have a bad stomach ache. Go to church without me; I shall be fine."

"Art thou certain, son?" asked Thomas' mother, concerned.

"Quite certain," Thomas answered, with a hint of pain, "I do not wish for you to miss church on my account."

Thomas had never been caught in a lie, so naturally his parents didn't question what he said. They each kissed him, saying, "We do hope that thou shalt soon feel better; we shall pray for thee. We shall return shortly." Hesitantly, they left for church. Soon after his parents left, Thomas felt a lot better. He rose up out of bed, got ready, and went to attend Lord Riley's event. Thomas felt bad about missing church, but felt destined to attend Lord Riley's spectacle due to the strange dream he had the night before.

On the way to the spectacle, Thomas heard Charles call his name from a short distance away. "Hey mate, wait! I shall go to church with thee." Thomas cringed, and ignored Charles. He walked faster as he thought, *"I do not wish to explain to Charles that I am going to Lord Riley's spectacle, lest I be called a hypocrite."*

Charles thought that Thomas was too far away to hear him, so he told his parents, "Pray, go ahead without me. I do see that Thomas is taking a different way to church. I shall go with him, and meet you there." His parents smiled and waved at their son as Charles ran after Thomas shouting, "Hey mate, wait! Dost thou not hear?"

Thomas cringed and stopped, thinking, "Oh no. How am I going to explain to Charles that I will be attending Lord Riley's bloody spectacle, especially after all the bad things I said to him about it?"

Charles soon caught up with Thomas, putting his hands down to his knees and gasping for air. "What is wrong?" he asked. "Hast thou lost thy hearing? Or art thou plainly ignoring me?"

Thomas stuttered, trying to avoid Charles' question because he didn't want to lie or hurt Charles' feelings. "Oh, hi-aw-Charles, aw-why dost thou not go to church with thy parents?"

Baffled, Charles responded, "Ah, excuse me, I am going to church today with thee, foolish lad! Didst thou not hear me shout? I was not that far away."

Thomas walked with a look of guilt on his face as he answered, "Charles, thou art me mate. I do not wish to hurt thy feelings. However, I prefer that thou dost go to church with your parents today."

Flabbergasted at hearing this, Charles responded, "What dost thou mean, thou dost not wish to hurt me feelings? Thou hast never before acted so strangely!" Thomas stopped at the junction of two roads; one road led to church and the other led to the arena where Lord Riley was holding his event. Charles started walking down the road leading to church, but stopped, noticing that Thomas wasn't walking. "Well, art thou not going to answer me question on our way to church?" Thomas looked down at the ground, glancing at the other road, the one that did not lead to church, while taking a deep breath. As his cheeks filled with air, he looked like a chipmunk. Seeing this look on Thomas' face, Charles knew that he was definitely hiding something. It didn't take Charles long to figure out what, by the way Thomas kept glancing at the road that didn't lead to church. Charles began laughing. "Oh no! Pray do not tell me that the very same fellow who said 'I shall never, ever, in my whole life attend one of those bloody spectacles', is actually going to attend one and break the Sabbath!"

Thomas put his right hand over his eyes. "Heaven help me. For indeed, I do deserve the words that I hear." He turned towards Charles. "I am sorry, mate. There is no time for explanations. Though I do not desire to attend the fight of Dare's brother, I must." Thomas started walking down the road that lead to the fight.

Baffled, Charles gave a twist of his head. "Halt! What dost thou mean, no time for explanations? Thou art not the same Thomas that I know." Charles jogged to catch up. He stopped Thomas by putting both hands on his shoulders. Charles stared into Thomas' eyes, "Hearken, if thou dost see Dare's brother fight today, so shall I, and there is nothing that thou canst say to change my mind. Therefore, thou might as well tell me what made thee change thy mind about attending Lord Riley's spectacle?"

Thomas looked away from Charles' stare, putting his hands over his eyes he shook his head, knowing that there was no way he could talk Charles out of following him. Even if he could, Charles would always consider him to be a hypocrite. Therefore, Thomas explained his whole dream to Charles on their way to the fight. Very amused by Thomas' dream, Charles asked,

"Tell me, dost thou not believe that this dream may have been merely a bad nightmare?"

Annoyed by the knowledge that Charles was thinking him mad, Thomas answered, "Charles, I do know that this dream sounds like the ravings of a madman, but God works in mysterious ways. I truly believe God sent an angel to me in my dream last night, convincing me to attend Lord Riley's spectacle."

"Why? For what purpose?" Charles asked, unconvinced.

"I do not know yet." Thomas answered, even more annoyed.

"Alright, what ever thou dost say," Charles said, rolling his eyes and thinking, "God, help me mate to not go mad!"

# CHAPTER XXII
# BULL BAITING EVENT SETS ATTENDANCE RECORD

When Thomas and Charles arrived at the fight, they saw thousands of people. This was by far a record attendance for bull baiting. Lord Riley had taken bull baiting to the next level. People were waiting in line for several hours just to get in. Thomas and Charles waited patiently in line. As they slowly approached the entrance, they heard some people complain the event was extremely over priced. Along with several other people, they had not known how much the event would cost because it had not been announced. Thomas and Charles didn't think much about this until they were almost at the entrance, and saw several people turn around and leave because of the price of the event.

Thomas was now concerned about the price, and tugged at the coat of the man in front of them, inquiring. "Excuse me, good sir, exactly how much money is admission to this event?"

"Nine shillings a person," the man answered, with a slight chuckle, for he was thinking, *"There is no way these lads will be able to afford this fight."* The price of admission was over four times the amount of money that Lord Riley normally charged.

Thomas and Charles exchanged shocked looks as Thomas said, "I do not have half that amount of money on me. Even though it seemed so real, I suppose that what I had last night was just what thou didst said it was, a bad nightmare." Thomas sulked for a second, then perked up, remembering the amount of money that Charles had received from Lord Riley. "That is, unless of course, thou didst bring the money Lord Riley gave thee, mate."

Charles shook his head no, and said, "Sorry mate." He paused, putting his hand on Thomas' shoulder and attempting to console him. "But consider the bright side. If we do not attend, thou wilt not break thy word about never attending a bull bating event."

"Thou art right," Thomas replied, discouraged. "Let us leave."

As Thomas started to walk away, Charles suddenly remembered something, "Wait," he mumbled quietly, "The pouch that I grabbed this morning was the wrong one." Charles reached into his pocket to check. Sure enough, he had accidentally grabbed the pouch containing ten shillings and thirty-two pence, instead of his pouch that contained only forty-four pence that he was taking to church to tithe. Suddenly feeling less skeptical, Charles called to Thomas, "Come here."

Thomas turned around and walked towards Charles answering, "Yes?"

Charles handed Thomas all his money, saying, "For the first time, I do begin to believe that there may be some truth to thy dream."

Thomas also pulled out his own money and counted sixty-four pence. They had just enough money to enter. "I knew that an angel visited me last night. I knew it," Thomas said confidently. Soon they were just seconds away from the entrance. That was when Thomas read a discouraging sign that said, "No young ones allowed, unless accompanied by guardian." With just a few seconds to react, Thomas tugged again on the coat of the man in front of him. "Pardon me, would you be so kind as to do us a favor?"

The man saw the money in Thomas' hand and read the sign. Knowing exactly what Thomas was going to ask of him, the man answered, "Certainly. What may I have the pleasure of doing for thee, young master?"

Thomas held the money up to the man asking, "Pray, say that we are with you, so we can attend this event."

The man quickly grabbed the money out of Thomas' hand. "Of course, young master," the man answered in a skeptical tone. "Fret not, for I give my word." The man put the money in his left coat pocket, then turned around, paid the ticket taker nine shillings, then quickly darted inside.

Thomas shouted out, "WAIT! What about us? You did give your word!" The man ignored Thomas as he kept walking rapidly, with a fiendish smirk on his face. Thomas and Charles had security holding them back and preventing them from chasing after the man.

At that moment, Vivian was close by with his uncle, Lord Riley. Vivian heard Thomas yell, then turned and saw him. Vivian was surprised, and tugging on his uncle's sleeve, he pointed at Thomas and Charles, saying, "What the bloody hell! I declare! 'Tis Thomas and Charles! What draws those bloody bastards here?" Lord Riley turned around and looked at them with a fiendish smile. Immediately he signaled his guards to stop the man that Thomas and Charles were pointing and yelling at. Lord Riley's guards grabbed the man just before he got lost in the crowd. Next, Lord Riley signaled his guards to bring the man over to Thomas and Charles. Seeing this, Vivian rubbed his hands with a big smile, for he thought, *"Boy, this is going to be great! Thomas and Charles are now going to be humiliated by my uncle in front of all these people."* Much to Vivian's dismay, his uncle was greatly pleased at seeing Thomas and Charles. He walked over to them with a closed-lipped smile. Both lads had looks on their faces which read, "Oh no! We're in trouble now." Much to their surprise, Lord Riley ordered his guards to remove their hands from them at once.

"Master Thomas, what seems to be thy problem?" Lord Riley asked with apparent concern.

As he pointed at the man he had given his money to, Thomas hesitantly answered, "I gave this man ten shillings and ninety-six pence to pay the admission for myself and Charles, but instead of paying for us, he put the money in his left coat pocket and kept it for himself, breaking his word."

Vivian quickly butt in, "Oh poor bloody babies. Ye should go crying home to your bloody mo-"

Lord Riley interrupted Vivian with a backhanded slap in the chest, scolding him, "Shut thy mouth! Leave us at once."

Vivian responded with a droopy face, "But uncle, I want to see the entrance of the Queen and Princess. Soon they shall arrive."

Lord Riley raised his hand at Vivian again as Vivian cringed. "Perhaps I was not clear! Go to thy seat! Stay there until the fight. Otherwise, I shall send thee home to thy sick father, whom thou shouldst be tending regardless, rather than being here." Vivian's father was really sick. Vivian pictured being at home, watching his father vomiting on the floor and having to clean it up. Knowing that his uncle wasn't bluffing, he turned and gave Thomas and Charles a jealous, angry look. With his face still black and blue, from Thomas' beating he walked to his seat. As Vivian was leaving, Lord Riley glared at the man he had stopped, and asked, "'Tis true that you did break your word, and did steal my friends' money?"

Trembling with fear, the man answered, "No my Lord, the young lads are mistaken."

With a heavily raised voice, Lord Riley argued, "So in other words, you are calling my friends liars?"

The man babbled out, "Uh-uh-no My Lord, I-just think they-uh-were-mistaken, uh-yah! That is it, mistaken."

Lord Riley turned, stretched out the puppy he was holding towards Thomas asking, "Would you be so kind as to hold my pup."

"Certainly," Thomas answered. His baffled look remained as he took the pup.

Lord Riley looked towards the man's full coat pocket, as the man began trembling with fear. "If I reach in your coat pocket, shall I find money there?"

Sweat now poured down the face of the man, who was intensely afraid. His lips shook frantically up and down as he answered, "I am not certain, my lord."

Lord Riley asked again, this time yelling, "Yea or nay, shall I find any money there?

The terrified man did not answer, but began to shake as if he were having a seizure. Lord Riley instructed his guard to hold the man while he searched the man's left pocket. "Indeed there is money here." Lord Riley said sounding unsurprised. "In fact it feels like ten shillings and ninety-six pence, exactly." Lord Riley pulled the money out of the man's coat pocket and counted it. "What a coincidence! I am right! I must be a soothsayer!" Lord Riley held the money up, looking at the people in line and asking loudly, "Was there anyone here who did see this man take money from these two fine lads?"

Three people who had been directly in back of Thomas and Charles answered, "Yes,"

"We did."

"The man even gave his word that he would pay for them."

Lord Riley had security write down the names of the persons that testified. "Thanks for helping out," Lord Riley said to the three who testified, and let them in for free. Lord Riley turned back to the man, glaring at him and shaking his head, "Our law states that you shall be found guilty upon the testimony of two or more witnesses."

Upon hearing this, the man turned and tried to run away, but the guards quickly tackled and held him. Lord Riley walked up to the man, and looked down upon him with narrowed eyes. He whispered so Thomas and Charles couldn't hear. "I am certain you are fully aware that the consequence for stealing is having your hands chopped off?" Lord Riley turned to his guards. "Take this thief away; have it be done."

The thief was dragged away, screaming for mercy, "No, my Lord! I beg of you!" Lord Riley ignored the screams, and turned around with a huge smile as he walked up to Thomas and Charles to shake their hands. Both looked flabbergasted, and wondered why Lord Riley was being so nice to them. Lord Riley's reasoning was they had two spectacular dogs that he wanted to use for breeding. Lord Riley thought that if he could get these two lads to enjoy themselves today and become bull-baiting fans, he could influence them to breed their dogs with his, after all. After Lord Riley shook hands, he handed the lads all of their money back, saying, "It pleases me greatly to see the change of heart ye two have had in deciding to attend one of my events. Ye two shall be treated like royalty today."

Right after Lord Riley said this, a voice shouted, "Make way for the Queen." Lord Riley, along with everyone around, bowed humbly, for Queen Mary had just arrived.

# CHAPTER XXIII
# BLOODY MARY LIVES UP TO
# HER NAME

When not wearing a stern expression, Queen Mary was very attractive, with a slender figure and long, light brown hair. The Queen was passionate and had a burning desire to bear children. The fact that she never did drove her to the verge of insanity, engendering an unquenchable wrath. Queen Mary was greatly feared, so much in fact that she was given the famous nickname, "Bloody Mary." More people were burned at the stake and had their heads chopped off at her command than any other king or queen ever, including her fierce father, King Henry VIII.

With his head still humbly bowed, Lord Riley addressed the Queen. "Welcome, your most gracious majesty! It brings me great honor that thou hast decided to attend one of my events. I shall cherish for all of eternity your royal presence here today."

Queen Mary sighed, thinking, *"Hoopla, hoopla! Here we go again, more rump kissing, although, this Lord Riley is the biggest rump kisser of all."*

Noticing that the Queen was looking at the pup in Thomas' arms, Lord Riley raised his head. "I have a gift for your highness. 'Tis with extreme pleasure that I present you with little Moe. His sire is Terror, the best dog that I have ever owned. You have my word, he shall grow up to make an outstanding guard dog for the royal family." As Lord Riley was talking, the Queen's younger half sister, Princess Elizabeth, and her cousin Vadra ran over to Thomas and the pup. Both young ladies were great beauties and had perfect figures. Princess Elizabeth had long red hair with pretty curls. Vadra had brown eyes and curly, dark brown shoulder-length hair to match. The Princess smiled as Thomas bowed his head in respect to her. Princess Elizabeth laughed joyfully as she petted and kissed the pup on the lips; the pup reciprocated and licked the Princess in turn. The pup felt the Princess' great love towards him and loved her every bit and more back.

Lord Riley went to take the pup out of Thomas' hands and place into the hands of the Princess, but as he reached for the pup, the Queen stopped him abruptly. "Halt! What makes you so certain that we shall accept this pup? We already have fine royal guard dogs!"

Lord Riley pondered looking at the Princess. She had a huge smile on her face as she kissed the puppies' face. Lord Riley thought, *"If the Queen does not accept this pup, Princess Elizabeth will bawl like a baby, and become angry with the Queen, in which case the Queen, in turn, shall become angry with me, which will surely mean, off with my head!"* Lord Riley bowed humbly. "Pray have mercy, your most gracious majesty, if my gift offends you."

The Queen looked at little Moe thinking, *"This indeed is a nice looking pup. I am sure he shall make a great royal guard dog. Besides, he surely does bring great joy to the Princess."* The Queen took out a sword, pulled it out of its sheath, and walked over to Lord Riley, the sword in her right hand and the sheath in her left. Seeing the Queen walking towards him, Lord Riley kept his head bowed, though he was shaking with fright because he thought that the Queen was dissatisfied with the pup as a gift and was moments away from personally chopping off his head. The Queen held the sword and sheath above Lord Riley's head. Lord Riley's eyes were closed tight and tears poured down his face over his quivering lips.

He was just about to scream, "I beg of your royal highness! Pray have mercy upon me!" But much to his pleasant surprise, the Queen said, "Your noble gift is gladly accepted." (Lord Riley opened his eyes and slowly raised his head.) "Therefore, I present you with this Royal sword, which bears my insignia on the blade." After showing Lord Riley the insignia, the Queen put the sword back into its sheath, and the nearby crowd was awed by the splendor of this gift. Not hearing applause, Queen Mary glanced at the crowd, annoyed. Seeing her glance, the people knew what she wanted, and they whistled and cheered for their lives. Cheers followed from the rest of the crowd. However, nobody was cheering sincerely for Lord Riley because they felt robbed by the outrageous ticket prices.

Upon accepting the Queen's gift, Lord Riley kept his head bowed and acted as if his tears of fear were tears of joy. "Many thanks, your most gracious majesty. Your generous gift has made this the happiest moment of my life." Lord Riley said with his shirt soaked by tears of fear. Again, there was no applause until the Queen glanced at the crowd.

The Queen turned to look at Thomas with a smile, saying, "Go ahead; you may present the Princess with the pup."

As Thomas did so, he bowed saying, "My Princess, it brings me great joy to present you with this wonderful pup." The Princess kissed Thomas on his cheek as she received the pup. This pleased the Queen. She nodded and smiled again at Thomas. The Queen naturally thought Thomas and Charles were Lord Riley's sons because they were both standing next to him and Thomas was the one who presented the Princess with little Moe.

The Queen asked, "What are your names, young lords?" Thomas and Charles smirked, for they were not lords. They bowed, telling the Queen only their first names. Afterwards, the royal family started walking to their seats. The Queen stopped and looked at Thomas and Charles, who remained standing in the same spot, saying, "Well, do not just stand there! Ye two shall attend today's event with the Royal family. Come now."

Hearing this, Thomas and Charles smiled and replied, "Our humble thanks, your most gracious majesty." Then they ran up to Princess Elizabeth and Vadra, who were waiting for them with smiles.

A few moments later, the man who had tried to steal Thomas and Charles' money momentarily escaped from the guards, and ran close to the Queen before he was tackled again.

The Queen stopped as she asked Lord Riley, "What was this man's transgression?"

As he answered the Queen, Lord Riley looked annoyed at his guard for allowing the thief to make a scene. "He tried to steal Thomas and Charles' mo-."

The Queen's eyes filled with rage. She raised her hand, preventing Lord Riley from saying another word. The two young lads had already found favor with her. "No need to hear anymore!" The Queen turned to her head knight, pointed at the thief, and commanded, "Off with his head!"

At this moment, Thomas and Charles were playing with little Moe while talking to Princess Elizabeth and Vadra. They didn't pay close attention to what the Queen had just said. With a dazed look Thomas asked, "What did the Queen just say?"

Princess Elizabeth answered with a smile. "The Queen said, off with his head!"

Thomas and Charles thought that was what she had said. Thomas quickly turned around in an effort to save the thief, but was too late. The head knight's sword was already in motion. Thomas and Charles witnessed the thief's head being chopped off before their eyes. Thomas had his mouth open and was just about to ask "Why?" When Lord Riley wisely put his hand over Thomas' mouth preventing him from questioning the Queen.

Lord Riley kept Thomas' mouth covered and whispered in his ear, "Hold thy tongue foolish lad. There is nothing anyone can do now for that pitiful thief. Do not insult the Queen's decision, lest we be beheaded also!" Lord Riley made sense. Thomas held his tongue as he watched the man's body squirm around without a head. Thomas and Charles, with flabbergasted expressions, looked at the Princess and Vadra. The young ladies' big beautiful smiles remained undisturbed as they continued to pay attention to little Moe as if nothing had happened. This was an everyday routine to the Princess and to Vadra. Lord Riley, noticing the lads' flabbergasted expressions, snapped his fingers to signal his servant Brent, who was serving wine. Brent speedily came over and held his wine tray in front of the Queen, keeping his head bowed. The Queen accepted the offer and with a slight nod, took a glass from his tray. Thus acknowledged, Brent then turned his tray towards Lord Riley, who bowed his head and took three glasses, handing one each to Thomas and Charles.

"Drink," Lord Riley told them, "This shall calm the nerves."

Seeing wine being served, the Princess wanted to drink also. With a raised finger, she signaled Brent. "Over here." Brent gulped, looking at the Queen.

Her eyes read, "Wise choice to look at me first." With a slight smile and nod, the Queen acknowledged it was all right.

With a relieved smile, Brent gladly rushed over to the Princess and Vadra and served them wine. The Princess and Vadra enjoyed their wine while sharing their opinions with Thomas and Charles. Due to the image fresh in their minds of the headless man squirming around, Thomas and Charles were oblivious to everything being said. They sipped their wine, nodding their heads and acting as if they were paying attention to all that was said. When they were finished drinking, Lord Riley offered them another glass.

"Yes! Please my Lord." Charles responded without hesitation.

Lord Riley signaled Brent, and allowed the Queen to take another glass first, before taking three more glasses, handing the two lads one glass each. Lord Riley commended them, patting them on the shoulders, "Now that's the spirit! These events are always full of excitement! Ye two young masters are always more than welcome to attend, for free of course, anytime ye desire." Lord Riley knew they were troubled by seeing the thief executed. He attempted to make light of the matter in order not to upset them or discourage them from attending his events in the future. After drinking their second cup of wine, Thomas and Charles, along with the Queen and Princess, were escorted by the royal family knights to their seats.

As they walked in, the whole place rose from their seats in respect, repeatedly shouting, "God save the Queen!"

With narrowed eyes and a frown, Vivian bowed along with the crowd. He was breathing very heavily as he watched the royal family's entrance, and was very much more jealous than before, for he witnessed Thomas seated right next to the Princess and sniffed the wine from their breaths as they passed.

With a smile, Lord Riley sat next to Vivian and put his arm around him. "I do declare, this is a special moment indeed, one that I am certain that thou, like me, shalt cherish for the rest of thy life. For behold! Directly in front of us sit the Queen and Princess!" Vivian didn't respond. Instead, he sank low in his seat with arms crossed, sulking as he watched Thomas, Charles, Vadra and the Princess exchange stories and laughter. He was fully aware that he could have been the one sipping wine and sitting next to the beautiful Princess, if only he had kept his big mouth shut, and had not pointed out Thomas and Charles to his uncle.

# CHAPTER XXIV
# BLOODY SUNDAY

An opera singer sang a song in the Queen's honor, then the event began. Lord Riley had his normal routine for the opening event. A bull was chained to a stake. Five dogs were soon to be released, one at a time. Thomas watched the chaining of the bull. Knowing what was soon to come, he excused himself to go to the privy. The Princess looked at Thomas with a smile, telling him as he walked away, "You are excused. However, you shall not be excused should you miss any of the event with me."

Seeing Thomas leave looking ill and knowing his feelings towards bull bating, Vivian seized the moment. He patted Charles on the shoulder and whispered in his ear, "Greetings mate." (Charles listened with a sour expression.) "'Twould not be proper to have the seat next to the Princess vacant during the event. Therefore, if for some unfortunate reason, Thomas is unable to return before the fight, 'twould be proper for me to be invited to take his place."

Charles stood, and turned, whispering in reply, "If you are invited, it shall have to

come from the Princess, for I shall not betray me mate!" Charles then excused

himself to the royal family.

On Thomas' way to the privy, he considered the spectacle that was about to occur, and the pressure that now bore upon him from the Princess. He vomited the moment he walked in the privy, then, he wiped his face and prayed, "Lord God, what purpose is there for me to be here?" Thomas stayed in the privy, with no intention returning to his seat before the spectacle was over.

Charles soon came in, shaking his head at Thomas. "Thomas, thou art being very disrespectful to the Queen and royal family. I know thou dost hate to watch bull baiting; however thou must, lest thou insult the Princess and royal family, incurring their wrath." With a bitter frown on his face, Charles paused for a second before continuing, "And we both do know what the Queen is capable of doing when brought to wrath!"

"My regrets, Charles. I can not go back!"

"Didst thou not hear the Princess say that there will be no excuse if thou miss any of the event?" Thomas breathed heavily and did not answer. "Do thou consider the humiliation the Princess shall bear if her escort should abandon her." Thomas remained silent, breathing even heavier. "So be it. Thou art alone in this," Charles said, walking towards the exit, paused, then turned around and sarcastically added, "Fret not about the Princess' feelings; Vivian shall comfort her. Being a gentleman, he hath offered to take your chair, next to hers. Nor shouldst thou concern thyself about any consequences. I am most certain that Vivian shall only speak kind words on thy behalf." With that, Charles left the privy.

These words made Thomas tremble with fear. Nor did he wish to hurt the feelings of the Princess. Sitting next to her was a once in a lifetime opportunity, the kind of opportunity most people like Vivian only dream about. Thomas soon gathered himself together and left the privy. Charles was outside, waiting with a smile. "I knew thou wouldst have a change of heart," he said as they walked back to their seats. They arrived the moment the first dog, Golem, was released.

Seeing Thomas return, Vivian cringed mumbling, "Damn it!" With a forced smile, Thomas stood next to the Princess. She smiled back, handing little Moe to him as she stood up to cheer Golem. The bull swung his head from side to side while maintaining eye contact with Golem. Golem sprawled back, his body swaying ever so slightly with anticipation a few feet in front of the bull. The moment the bull's head swayed near the ground, Golem attacked. He lunged, locking his jaws on the bull's nose. Golem held on for three minutes before being thrown thirty feet into the air, due to a piece of nose flesh being torn off the bull. Then the second dog, Balgar, was released. Balgar attacked in the same way. Four minutes later, Golem slowly rose to his feet, staggering back to the bull as Golem was thrown twenty-five feet into the air, due to more flesh being torn off the bull's nose. The third dog, Dagger, was then released. Smelling fresh blood flowing, Dagger charged, without pacing, straight for the bull's nose and locked on, while Golem attacked the throat. Six minutes later, more flesh was torn off the bull as both dogs were tossed twenty feet into the air. Balgar had now risen to his feet, and lunged, again locking on the bull's nose as the fourth dog, Red Rage, was released. Red Rage came charging out, biting the torn flesh from the bull's throat. Dagger soon joined in, helping by biting the bull on the left side near the heart area. Golem was unable to rise. Determinedly, he crawled over, but was not able to be any help. As the other three dogs held on, blood from the bull quickly began to gush all over the place as the crowd mercilessly erupted with cheers. Several minutes later, the bull's nose was more than half torn off as Balgar was tossed into the air again. This time he landed badly injured. The fifth dog, Ugly Jack, was then released. He charged, locking onto the bull's nose, and soon drove the bull's face into the ground, while Dagger and Red Rage tenderized the bull's flesh.

Lord Riley, who was directly in back of Thomas, bent over, putting his hands on Thomas' shoulders and commenting, "See? This is not so bad, son. Notice how my dogs are destroying the bull? This is what God created them to do, kill!"

Hearing this, Thomas kept a phony smile on his face but trembled slightly with rage. On the inside, he just wanted to explode and sweep Lord Riley's hands off of him, while screaming at the top of his lungs, *"Do not ever call me son! You are not my father! These dogs may have been created to kill, but not to sacrifice their lives for people's sick amusement!"*

The bull soon breathed his last breath, and the crowd erupted with even louder cheers. Balgar and Golem were taken away in the back where nobody was permitted to enter.

Lord Riley called, "Owen, come here."

"Yes, milord," Owen responded, immediately going to Lord Riley.

Lord Riley motioned with his index finger for Owen to put his ear next to his mouth. Lord Riley then whispered. "Balgar and Golem will probably be dead by morning. Even if they survive, their injuries are too severe for them to be any use to me again. Therefore, take them to the bloody cage in the back and do them a favor."

"I know milord, off with their heads!"

"SHHH," (Lord Riley stressed) "When you pass by the guards, remind them to make bloody sure that nobody, and I mean nobody is permitted back there. Understand?"

Owen took a shilling tip out of Lord Riley's hand. "Yes, milord. Once again I shall remind them," Owen responded, then turned and left. Thomas' excellent hearing allowed him to overhear what had been said. This made him feel nauseous. He held his head down to prevent himself from vomiting again.

Vivian, noticing Thomas in this state, bent over and sarcastically whispered to him, "Oh, is this too unbearable to handle? Perhaps vomiting in front of the royal family and on the Princess shall make you feel much better! If I were you, I would spare myself the embarrassment by going home!"

After hearing this derogatory comment, the ill feeling in Thomas' stomach subsided. He looked at Vivian, and whispered back with anger. "You would love that, would you not? Therefore you could take my place, having this once in a lifetime opportunity to put your vile black and blue face next to the Princess!" Thomas paused with a smile, "I am feeling much better, thanks to you. Therefore, I shall remain!"

Vivian leaned back in his seat, grimacing again. Throwing a fist across his body he said, "Damn it!"

The three dogs that survived were permitted to tear the bull apart for their reward, consuming as much flesh as they could for ten minutes, before their bloody faces were pulled away from the bull. Afterwards, the dogs were taken out of the arena by a different way than the injured dogs prior to them. When the dogs were gone, twenty men ran to the bull, carrying it off as Lord Riley walked towards the center of the arena. His shoes squished from all the blood shed on the ground. When he arrived at the center, he clapped his hands together with a big phony smile. "Let us here some cheers for me wonderful dogs!" he said as the crowd stood up, cheering. At first, Thomas did not stand up, until Charles nudged him and made him stand up and applaud. Lord Riley motioned for the crowd to be quiet. "If ye think that was something, ye shall be astonished at what ye are about to behold! For the first time ever in this sport, ye shall witness a dog attempting to kill an enormous unchained bull all by himself. I would not think this would be possible, had I not witnessed it with me own eyes, by the brother of the dog which ye are about to behold. This incident happened by accident, when a young master who is like a son to me, who is sitting over there next to the Queen and princess," (as Lord Riley said this, he pointed at Thomas and bowed to the Queen. The Queen looked confused as she bowed in return, for she thought Thomas was Lord Riley's son) "was soon to feel deaths sting! He would have if not for the brother of the dog ye shall soon behold had not come to his rescue by killing the bull!" The crowd applauded. The Princess clapped, smiling as she looked at Thomas, whose eyes were closed as he shook with rage, his face bright red. Thomas distinctly remembered that moment when Lord Riley watched him nearly die, without lifting a bloody finger to help.

The Princess, concerned by Thomas' expression, nudged him while continuing to clap. "Are you alright young master? Your face is brighter than the color of my hair"

Thomas answered, putting on a phony smile. "Yes, quite fine, my Princess. I am just overwhelmed to be in the presence of the Royal Family!"

Amused with Thomas' facial expression, the Princess replied, "Silly lad," while rolling her eyes towards him with a smile and slight shake of the head.

After the applause, Lord Riley continued, "In addition, the dog ye will soon behold hath had ninety-nine fights to the death against the best fighting dogs in the world. He hath never tasted defeat, and has suffered only minor injuries. In celebration of bout number one hundred, he faces the most challenging foe of all. For behold, over to me left, Enormous Elias! (Lord Riley shouted the bull's name while pointing back stage as a curtain was opened, exposing Elias. The crowd was awed by Elias' enormous size and bulging muscles.) Strongest of the bulls, Elias also hath never tasted defeat, and is a creature worthy of taking on a lion." Lord Riley quieted the crowd to a dead silence with his hands, looked at the drummer and gave a nod of his head. The drummer, in turn, immediately gave a drum roll. "Your Royal Highness, Lords and Ladies. Without any further ado, it is my great pleasure to introduce the fiercest, best damn bloody fighting dog in the world. Me very own (a two second pause as he caught his breath, before an echoing scream) "THE LEGENDARY TERROR!!!!" Terror was released the instant Lord Riley screamed out his name. He came running out into the arena, smelling the blood from the earlier fight. He paced around the arena like a hungry caged lion, while keeping eye contact with Elias, snarling, and growling all the while. He overflowed with rage, knowing full well that they were just moments away from a bloody fight to the death. The bloodthirsty crowd roared it's loudest, knowing the fight was about to begin.

The Princess yelled, cheering and holding little Moe over the rail. "Behold thy powerful father, little Moe, whom thou shalt soon resemble."

Thomas looked at Terror in disbelief, saying to Charles, "That is not me dog's brother out there, for unlike Dare, he has no kindness in him."

Charles patted Thomas on the shoulder and replied, "In flesh and blood, not in spirit. All kindness in his being was destroyed for good, ninety-nine fights ago."

Lord Riley soon darted out of the arena as Elias was released. He was much bigger and stronger than the bull in the previous fight. Elias circled around the arena, staring into Terror's eyes, while each created a cloud of dust. Elias soon charged at Terror, who held still until the last fraction of a second. That's when Terror dodged out of the way, avoiding Elias like a matador. Elias circled around again, as both animals kept their eyes locked on one another. Elias soon charged again at Terror. Again, Terror dodged away at the last fraction of a second. This time, when Elias missed, he took his eyes off of Terror for a fraction of a second. That's when Terror sprung into the air, locking his enormous and powerful jaws on Elias nose, hanging on for dear life. Witnessing this, the crowd erupted louder than ever in the history of the sport or the arena.

An awful lot of money had been bet on this match before the fight. Most people bet Terror would be the first to die. Therefore, most of the crowd cheered for the bull to win by chanting, "Kill bull kill! Kill bull kill."

This really disturbed the Princess. Her pup had been sired by the dog in the ring. She became really upset, especially with a man a few rows in back of her who was screaming over and over at the top of his lungs "KILL, BULL, KILL! KILL, BULL, KILL!" The man was influencing others to chant along also. Princess Elizabeth looked at the Queen, glancing at the man a few rows back with a hurt look. The Princess hugged little Moe. A little tear trickled down onto little Moe as the man a few rows back continued to scream bad things about little Moe's father. The Queen looked at the man, motioning to her head guard with a hand across her throat. Her head guard automatically knew what the Queen wanted. Instantly he ran in back of the man the Queen had looked at, and chopped off his head as the man was laughing and screaming, "KILL, BULL, KILL!" After this happened, nobody within three hundred feet of the Queen cheered for the bull.

Terror kept his jaws locked onto Elias' nose, as Elias shook him all over the arena. A lot of the people in the first few rows had blood splattered on them from this fight. The Princess and Queen were about to be splattered by blood as well, but as the blood flew towards them, Thomas jumped in the way, intercepting the blood with his clothes, arms and face. None of the blood landed on either the Queen or the Princess. Thomas' action really pleased the Queen, so much so, in fact, that she handed him a royal emblem to show her appreciation. Thomas bowed down in thanks. When he arose, the Princess helped wipe some of the blood off of his face and clothes with her handkerchief. Thomas watched the fight a little while longer until he just couldn't take any more. Even though Terror was full of evil, he was still Dare's brother. Thomas felt very sad, watching Terror shaking violently in mid air. This was unbearable. He turned and looked the other way, as he held himself back from crying. Suddenly, Thomas had a dejá vu experience of his dream last night. He watched the same people moving in slow motion, yelling and cheering for the bull to win. He looked up to where the giant had been standing in his dream, but he didn't see him there, but where the giant had been standing in his dream he saw a moving white light. After Thomas saw this, everything around him returned to moving at normal speed again.

Terror was soon thrown into mid air, as over half of Elias' nose and bone had been torn off. Blood spurted straight up in the air from Elias' nose, like a garden hose fully turned on. The crowd was awed, seeing this, and became dead silent as Elias staggered, then soon became unable to stand. Hearing the silence, Thomas slowly turned and saw Terror hobbling painfully over to Elias' jugular vein. Terror paused, taking in a few deep breaths, gathering up all his strength, before biting and ripping out the vein, just as his brother Dare had done when he fought and killed Bulldread. Even more thick blood began to spurt up into the air, resembling a giant fountain. The crowd remained quiet and in awe from the spectacle. They heard Elias scream out in agony as he took his last breath. When the blood from Elias stopped gushing, all eyes turned towards Terror, who was badly injured but victorious.

# CHAPTER XXV
# MARKED FOR DEATH

Immediately following the death of Elias, Vivian left with a perturbed expression on his face. He felt that it should have been him seated next to the Princess, rather than Thomas. After all, it was his uncle's event. The crowd quietly remained, still in awe. A huge smile filled Lord Riley's face as he walked into the center of the arena. He had bet more than half his riches on Terror at thirty-seven to one. He looked at Lord Edward, who had his hand on his head as he shook it back and forth in disbelief. Lord Edward felt furious stares upon him from his comrades, for they had believed him when he had guaranteed a victory over Terror. Several of them had also bet half their riches on Elias. Lord Riley was now undoubtedly the richest lord in England. Changing his smile to a grin, he looked at Terror, who softly howled in pain, begging for praise just once, before his life ended. Lord Riley ignored his dog's wishes. He looked into his dog's heart-shattered eyes, squinting with a closed smile as he mumbled, "What a bloody shame; I could have made even more money off of thee the next time. Unfortunately, thou art too bloody injured; thou wouldst only be a nuisance, if permitted to live." Lord Riley turned away from Terror, motioning for him to be carried in the back on a stretcher, then turned back with coarse, merciless eyes, "Thou art now obsolete." As Terror was being taken away, the crowd slowly began clapping, which was soon followed by an uproar. Terror had proven that he was a remarkable creature, with a heart more powerful than anything imaginable. Through his courage and the bloody mess, a few people's hearts were softened. Their attitudes towards the brutality of the sport changed and they would never attend such an event again. The Princess turned her face to Thomas' shoulder, shedding a tear of remorse as Terror was being carried away. As Thomas softly rubbed the back of her head comfortingly, he remembered how his uncle had snapped Dare's bones back into place. He also remembered his dream of last night. At that moment, Thomas knew the purpose of his being there. It was to try to save Terror from having his head chopped off.

Thomas told Charles, "I must attempt to save the life of Dare's brother."

Charles sighed before replying, "I am sorry, Thomas. There is nothing anyone can do for Dare's brother. He looks even worse than Dare did after he fought Bulldread."

Thomas rose up out of his seat, saying, "I do not believe that Dare's brother cannot be saved. Because of me dream last night, I believe his destiny is to live."

Charles also stood up as he replied, "Perhaps thou art right. I shall go with thee." Thomas was just about to say goodbye to the Princess when she rose with her pup in her arms. The Princess had overheard what Thomas and Charles had said.

"We shall come along also!" Princess Elizabeth firmly stated. "I care very much about the well-being of my pup's father."

Thomas was about to say, "'Tis probably better to remain, for you may see little Moe's father die."

As he started to speak, Charles grabbed his shoulder and whispered in his ear, "Let her come. Do not insult the Princess and create a spectacle, especially in front of the Queen."

Looking at the Princess, Thomas nodded his head. "Our thanks. We would be delighted to have you accompany us."

Princess Elizabeth saw a big sign where Terror was restrained which read. "No one allowed on the premises beyond this point." She knew that her two personal bodyguards, Hubert and Walter, would not let her out of their sight. They would also not permit her to walk back to where Terror was because of the sign. Hubert and Walter were trained to abide by rules.

The Princess whispered in Thomas' ear. "Go before me and Moe. We shall soon catch up." Thomas nodded his head to her, then both he and Charles bowed their heads to the Queen as they left to go help Terror. Shortly after they left, the Princess bowed to the Queen, excusing herself to go to the privy, and Hubert and Walter followed. Once the Princess had walked into the privy, she opened the side window and climbed out with Moe in her arms. She quickly slipped through the crowd to go meet up with Thomas and Charles, who at this time were trying to get past the exit where Terror was. They were restrained from going back there by a huge man named Donovan Harris, who was Lord Riley's head guard.

With his hands pushing against Thomas' and Charles' chests, Donovan gave them orders: "Halt! No one passes over this red line! Do you not see the sign?" Thomas looked at Donovan' huge hand pressed against his chest. He slowly lifted his eyes straight up, about seven feet, before making eye contact with Donovan.

Thomas gulped before answering, "Pray permit us to pass. I do believe that we can help Terror."

"A mad idea, lad!" Donovan chuckled as he replied, "Terror is too badly injured. Nobody can help him now."

Thomas kept facing straight up, keeping eye contact as he replied,

"'Twould be no harm in allowing us to tend to Terror. If you do not, Terror shall surely get his head chopped off!"

Donovan was surprised that Thomas knew this. Nobody was supposed to know that's what happens to the dogs that end up back there, for fear people who were opposed to bull baiting would have more grounds to use to outlaw the sport. Donovan attempted to play it off. "Who told you such a lie? Assuredly that shall not happen."

With his head still straight up in the air, and maintaining eye contact, Thomas shook his fist. "Do not play dumb nor lie! I know what goes on back there."

With his index finger, Donovan poked Thomas in the chest, and Thomas backed up. "Look, young lad! I do not give a bloody hell what you believe! We have strict orders to make bloody sure nobody gets past! (Donovan kept his finger pointed at Thomas as he said this.) Understand, little lad?"

"Thou didst hear the giant," Charles said, turning around. "I suppose that we should go say our goodbyes to the Queen and Princess."

Thomas, on the other hand, didn't budge. "Wait a moment, Charles. There is no more time to waste. These kind gentlemen shall let us pass!"

Thomas said this as he tried to walk past the guards. Upon crossing the red line, Donovan grabbed Thomas by the shirt collar and raised him in the air up to his face. With fury in his eyes, Donovan threatened, "Heed me warning little lad, leave at once; otherwise you shall see terror, if you pursue this matter any further, and it shall not be the dog." Donovan, along with the guards, chuckled at what he had just said.

At that moment, the Princess appeared, with Moe in her arms and yelled, "Put my friend down at once, you big buffoon!"

Donovan put Thomas down immediately, bowing as he replied, and speaking in a frightened tone of voice. "Yes, my Princess." The Princess walked up to Donovan and pointed her finger in his face. "Nobody lays another hand on any of my friends without paying serious consequences."

Donovan kept his huge head bowed, as did all the guards, as he replied, "Please forgive me, my Princess. I did not know that these were your friends!"

Moe growled, feeling the tension. While calming Moe with gentle strokes, the Princess replied with a stern look. "I will forgive you this time, if permitted to pass at once!"

Donovan kept his head bowed, closed his eyes, and took a deep breath, knowing he was in a bad dilemma. "Pray do understand, my Princess. I have been given the strictest of orders not to permit any one past this red line."

Princess Elizabeth laughed. "Ha, those orders have just been changed, lest I call the Queen to come here and remove your head!"

Hearing this, Donovan sweated with fear. "Once again, my apologies. I cannot let you pass."

The Princess turned around sharply. She stood still for a second before saying, "So be it! We shall pass that red line, and your head shall be chopped off in vain!" The Princess started walking towards Queen Mary yelling, "Oh-Que-!"

Waving his hands, Donovan quickly rose to his feet interrupting. "Permission hath been granted; you and your friends may pass the red line."

The Princess turned around sharply, with her head up high and holding her pup as she walked past the guards saying, "Wise choice. You shall live."

Donovan breathed very heavily, and was sweating as he bowed again. "My thanks, your Highness." (Donovan was the one who felt terror.)

Thomas knew that at any point, Lord Riley's servant could be a second away from chopping off Terror's head. Concerned, he said, "We must hurry. Terror doth not have much time!"

The Princess replied, "If that is the circumstance, then we shall separate. The first to find Terror shall alert the others by yelling, 'here lies Terror!'"

Thomas, uneasy with this plan, replied, "With all due respect, my Princess, your safety is of the utmost importance."

Annoyed, the Princess responded, lifting her hand and looking like the Queen, "There is no time for conflicts. Do as I say!"

Thomas and Charles were not about to question her anymore. They both bowed their heads to her, saying, "As you wish."

Thomas added, "If you are suspicious of anyone who may pose a threat, alert us at once."

With a smirk the Princess replied, "Worry not; such a fool does not exist,"

But a guard by the name of Genard Harper was, in fact, such a fool. Genard, seeing the Princess alone and vulnerable thought, *"'Tis my golden opportunity to become filthy rich, for I shall kidnap the Princess."* Genard turned to Donovan, his boss, who was still shaken up due to his confrontation with the Princess. "Begging leave to take a brief respite?"

"Permission granted."

"My thanks," Genard replied, consumed with greed. He walked fast in the same direction the Princess had walked. Once he was around a corner and out of everyone's sight, he ran and soon found the Princess. She was all by herself with Moe. Genard snuck up and grabbed her, while covering her mouth. Moe reacted instantly by biting Genard's hand. Genard released his hand over the Princess mouth for a second, as he shook it, shaking Moe off his hand and onto his leg.

But before he could replace his hand over her mouth, the Princess was able to scream out, "HELP!" Thomas heard the scream. Quickly, he ran over toward the direction of the sound of the Princess screaming, and saw Genard carrying her around a corner, with Moe latched on to his leg. Genard shook the leg that Moe was latched on to, trying to shake him off, but was unable to do so without using his hands. But if he did, the Princess would scream out longer and louder. So Genard cringed, dealing with the pain inflicted by Moe.

Thomas ran in back of them, keeping quiet and out of sight, for he knew that if Genard saw him, he would threaten the Princess' life, by saying something like, "Leave us, or the Princess' throat shall be sliced." Thomas played it smart, keeping close behind. He soon came across a large hammer and grabbed it.

Just when Genard was about to carry the Princess out of the arena through a deserted back exit door, Thomas ran up and smacked Genard in the back of the skull with the hammer. Genard, stunned, dropped to his knees while releasing the Princess. Genard grabbed his sword to pull it out, intending to kill Thomas and Moe. But the moment Genard had pulled it out, Thomas hit him again, this time even harder, in the back of the head. This knocked Genard out cold, and he hit the ground face first. Not knowing for sure that Genard was out cold, Thomas hit him yet again, to make certain that he was. This time he hit Genard as hard as he could on the right side of the temple. This hit ended Genard's life. Thomas, confident that Genard could do no more damage, helped the Princess up, making sure she was alright, which she was. The Princess, knowing Thomas had just saved her life, gave him a big kiss on the lips. Afterwards, she hugged him tight as she thanked him.

Thomas blushed, "The pleasure is mine, my Princess," Thomas said while holding her. After they held one another, they looked at Genard, whose face was drenched with blood from the blow to the temple and from Moe, who was now biting him on the nose.

The Princess bent down, feeling for a pulse, but felt none. She pulled Moe off of Genard. She wiped Moe's face clean of blood, placing him back in her arms, and looked up at Thomas like nothing very significant had happened. "Serves that bloody bastard right!" The Princess smiled and stood up as she continued, "Thou didst surely hit him hard. Thou must truly care for me."

Thomas put both hands over his eyes and shook his head from side to side. "Oh no! I just killed a man! Surely I shall hang!"

The Princess laughed. "That shall never happen, I promise! Thou shalt be a hero for this!" Thomas stared at Genard, exasperated as the Princess began to run, "Come at once! Let us find Terror." Not wanting the Princess out of his sight again, Thomas desperately tried to keep up, but fell a few steps behind because he was winded from chasing Genard and killing him. The Princess was the first to find Terror, just as Lord Riley's axe man, Owen, was moving his arm down to chop off Terror's head. Seeing this, the Princess quickly screamed, "HALT!" At this point, Owen would have ignored this command, but he saw the Princess out of the corner of his eye. He feared the Queen enormously. He tried to stop, but his momentum was too strong. He angled the axe to the right. The blade harmlessly scraped against Terror's left ear. In trying to avoid chopping off Terror's head, Owen ended up cutting the right side of his own outer thigh. Owen yelled out in pain, "Ouch!" Hearing the Princess scream and Owen yell, Charles came running over. They all walked into the cage where Terror was. The Princess put Moe down, and he went running over to his father, licking Terror's wounds and softly crying as if to say, "Do not give up, father; do not die." Thomas looked closely at Terror. He took his shirt off and ripped it into several pieces, and then wrapped the pieces around Terror's cuts to help stop the bleeding.

Charles ripped his shirt off too, and did likewise.

"Good work, Princess Elizabeth," Thomas complimented her. "You have saved Terror's life."

"Saved him," Owen replied with a puzzled look, as he wrapped the gash on his thigh with a cloth. "Forgive me for being so bold, my Princess. The kindest thing we can do for Terror is to put him out of his misery. He is too badly injured, and most likely he will be dead soon, regardless." Owen finished wrapping his cut as he stated, "Even if he miraculously survives, he would not have any kind of life."

The Princess stared at Owen with powerful gleaming eyes. "Silence! Do not interfere!"

Backing up, Owen gave short bows to her. "Yes, my Princess. I shall do as you say." Owen left to go find Lord Riley.

Terror was unconscious. The Princess and Charles calmly petted Terror on the shoulder and head.

Thomas carefully moved Terror onto his back, then felt Terror's neck to determine where it was out of place. When he found the spot, he looked up, closed his eyes, and quietly prayed. "If it be Thy will, help save me beloved dog's brother." After this prayer, Thomas snapped Terror's neck back in place perfectly, the way his uncle had taught him. Thomas then asked Charles and Princess Elizabeth to hold Terror still on his stomach as he carefully felt

Terror's spine. "I do not feel any broken bones. 'Tis a good sign," Thomas said, relieved. "However, I do feel two areas that are out of place." Once again, Thomas popped Terror's bones back in place as Charles and the Princess calmly petted Terror, whispering, "Tis alright, thou shalt be fine."

Terror was now slowly starting to gain consciousness. Thomas didn't have much time. He knew that once Terror gained full consciousness, he would attack them. Thomas acted quickly as he felt Terror's hips and shoulders. They were fine, except for the right shoulder, which was dislocated. Saying, "Now for the hard part," Thomas gently rolled Terror onto his left side, directing Charles and the Princess to hold Terror perfectly still. Thomas closed his eyes and took in a deep breath. Exhaling, he snapped Terror's shoulder back in place. Immediately afterward, Terror came to, howling in pain. Thomas grabbed the Princess and pulled her away from Terror as he tried to bite her. Charles grabbed little Moe, who was near his father's face at the time, and pulled him away. As Terror staggered to his feet attempting to kill them, they all got out of the dog's cage. Thomas shut the door on Terror's face, right after Charles had run out of the cage with little Moe. Terror stared at them, growling furiously.

# CHAPTER XXVI
# BLOODY MARY'S WRATH

Owen found Lord Riley, who at the time was entertaining the Queen with stories from his family's past about bull baiting. Owen attempted to get his attention by tapping him on the shoulder, but Lord Riley, enjoying the Queen's undivided attention, waved him off. Owen kept tapping on his shoulder, whispering, "Pray excuse the intrusion my Lord, but this matter is of the utmost importance!"

Lord Riley turned to Owen with a quiet snarl, saying, "For your sake, it had better be!"

Owen whispered in Lord Riley's ear what had happened, but not quietly enough to prevent the Queen from overhearing, for she was standing next to them. Quickly, the Queen turned to the privy where the Princess had gone. The Queen saw Hubert and Walter, both with horrified expressions on their faces.

As Walter searched through the crowd trying to spot the Princess, Hubert knocked on the privy asking, "Princess Elizabeth, are you within?"

The Queen, seeing this, screamed, "Hubert! Walter! Stand before me!!" Hubert and Walter approached the Queen, bowing and trembling with fear, as the Queen asked, "Do you two imbeciles know the whereabouts of Princess Elizabeth?" Hubert and Walter babbled in response. "Well?" asked the Queen.

Walter eventually managed to speak. "Have mercy! Your most gracious Majesty, we did escort Princess Elizabeth to the privy and kept a constant eye on the entrance. However, she never came out!"

The Queen slapped them both across their faces, "That is because she slipped through the window that ye two babbling buffoons were ignoring!" The Queen gave Hubert and Walter two seconds to respond. They froze, speechless. "If any harm comes to the Princess, chopping off your heads shall be merciful!" After the Queen scolded them, she turned to Owen, and shouted, "Bring me at once to the princess. Heads shall roll!" The Queen followed Owen, and was in turn followed by Lord Riley, Donovan and the Queen's royal knights, all trembled with fear. The Queen called out, "Princess Elizabeth! Where art thou?"

The Princess heard the Queen. She looked at Thomas' and Charles' bare chests. Knowing the Queen wasn't one that would listen to reason, she commanded, "Thomas, Charles, leave at once! There is no time to explain. Go!" Thomas and Charles heard the Queen just moments away. As they glanced at each other's bare chests, both immediately realized that the Queen would assuredly get the wrong idea. They turned, running for their lives, as the Queen and her knights walked around the corner, only to see Thomas and Charles fleeing with bare chests.

The Queen was shocked and her jaw dropped. Instantly she pointed at Thomas and Charles, screaming, "Off with their heads!" Five of the royal knights chased Thomas and Charles. Lord Riley, fearful lest he be held accountable, glared at his head guard as if to say, *"Why did you disobey my command by allowing them back here in the first place?"*

Princess Elizabeth bowed before Queen Mary, crying out. "Pray, spare their lives. They did nothing wrong. They only helped spare the life of my pup's father."

Lord Riley mumbled, "'Tis impossible." He looked in Terror's direction, and much to his surprise, saw Terror standing on all fours and taking a few steps. Terror growled because his shoulder was still sore, and soon lay down to rest on his uninjured side. Seeing this, Lord Riley quickly ran to Terror's cage, and felt the dog's bones. Finding none broken, Lord Riley was astonished. Clenching his hands he yelled, "YES!" He knelt down on his left knee, placed a hand on Terror's head, and whispered in his ear, "I am relieved indeed, knowing thou shall live, for soon thou shall fight again, making me even more filthy rich." Hearing this, Terror thought just before falling asleep, *"Why did those foolish kids not let me die? I would have been better off."* Terror had felt Thomas' healing hands of love upon him. It was the first time a human had ever showed kindness or love towards him. Terror felt very uncomfortable, not liking it. Thomas had sown seeds of love that day. But those seeds had no roots to cling onto, nor water. Terror's heart remained cold as ice, knowing that in his next fight, he would be used as a sacrifice.

Lord Riley walked out of Terror's cage, and approached the Princess, bowing as he said, "My thanks, Princess Elizabeth. Your majesty has saved the life of my best dog, for which I shall be eternally grateful."

Without looking, the Princess responded by quickly raising her hand. Then she began arguing with the Queen, "Perish thy thoughts you-"

Furiously, Queen Mary interrupted, "What am I supposed to think, when I see two young gentlemen caught with their shirts off, running away with guilt in their eyes? How could thee, Elizabeth? For thou hast brought great shame to the royal family! Why, I should . . ." (the Queen caught herself, and stopped short of saying "chop your head off").

Princess Elizabeth cried out, "Pray, look you at Terror and see the shirts of Thomas and Charles are wrapped around him. They did this to stop his bleeding. That is why they removed their shirts!"

The Queen calmed down a little, thinking, "'Tis a logical explanation." She questioned more, but in a calmer tone, "Oh! Pray tell, then, why did they run when they saw me arrive?"

"They ran, for I told them to do so."

"Why, then? Would it not be better to explain to me?"

"No!" Princess Elizabeth answered swatting a few tears away from her face. "You do not think logically. You are always quick in judging and ordering, OFF WITH THEIR HEADS! Thomas and Charles are perfect gentlemen. Furthermore, I do swear on the grave of our father, King Henry VIII, that nothing happened!"

Hearing these words, Queen Mary now had no doubts that her sister was telling the truth. So she changed the subject. "How dost thou dare to lie to thy guards and by stealth leave the privy through the window? Thou dost know 'tis not safe to go about without the guards. Thou couldst have been abducted or killed!" The Princess, in a crying tone, replied. "By faith, I am sorry. Pray believe me, I truly have learned my lesson! One of Lord Riley's guards did try to capture me . . ." (hearing this, the Queen had a shocked expression on her face) "and would have succeeded, had it not been for Thomas, who came to my rescue, killing the guard, and thus saving my life! For that, I owe Thomas my very life." Hearing this, the Queen knew that she had acted hastily, and that her sister would never forgive her if she were to shed the innocent blood of her hero. Lord Riley, who had overheard the conversation, gulped, and trembled with fear even more.

The Princess kissed little Moe on the head as she handed him to the Queen, saying, "Little Moe's father would also not be here right now had it not been for Thomas and Charles."

The Queen held little Moe in her arms, as little Moe licked her face. "'Tis too late!" said the Queen, looking away from Moe and holding her head up high with enormous pride. "Once I reach a decision, tis always final. Never have I reversed a decision."

The Princess, hearing this, ripped off the crown from her own head in rage. "If you do not reverse your decision, I shall never again address you as Queen! I shall also renounce my throne!" Shocked expressions came upon the faces of the royal guards. They all knew that if the Princess were anybody else, there would be no question that she would be burned at the stake, or worse, for what she had just said.

Meanwhile, Thomas and Charles had just been caught by two of the royal guards. They were dragged to the block that was used for beheading Lord Riley's badly injured dogs. One of the royal guards tied Thomas' hands behind him, and put Thomas' head on the bloodstained block, while

Sir Christopher, the Queen's chief guard, pulled out his sword and held it above his head. Sir Christopher was just about to bring it down, chopping off Thomas's head, when Thomas screamed out, "I rebuke thee, in Jesus' name!" Sir Christopher, with his sword raised above his head, could not move. It was almost as if an angel came down from heaven and stopped him. Thomas yelled again, "I rebuke thee, in Jesus' name!" Sir Christopher did not desire to chop off Thomas' head. Not only was Thomas still a young lad, but now God was brought into the picture. Sir Christopher knew, however, that if he disobeyed the Queen, his own head would be chopped off, along with that of Thomas and Charles. Therefore, Sir Christopher removed Thomas from the block momentarily, and had the mouths of both Thomas and Charles tied shut. Now neither of them could say another word.

As this was happening, the Princess kept crying and screaming her lungs out at the Queen. "If you do chop my good friends' heads off, never shall I speak to you again, nor shall I eat!" Princess Elizabeth was the closest thing to the daughter that the Queen so much desired. As the Princess bowed and cried out, the Queen looked at her with compassion. For the first time in her life, the Queen humbled herself. Turning to one of her royal guards, Sir Andrew by name, she commanded. "Go and find Sir Christopher, and tell him thus sayeth the Queen. Spare the young lads' lives."

Sir Andrew bowed answering, "At once, your most gracious Majesty." Then he ran, in an attempt to save Thomas and Charles' lives, who at that moment had their mouths tied shut. This time, Charles was put on the cutting board. His eyes bulged wide as he mumbled, with his face in blood of dogs that had been decapitated there.

With intense fear, Charles looked up at Sir Christopher out of the corner of his eye, and saw Sir Christopher's sword raised up in the air. Just as the sword was about to come down, chopping off Charles' head, Sir Andrew arrived yelling, "Halt! sayeth the Queen!" Sir Christopher immediately stopped, and put his sword back in its sheath. Sir Andrew bent over, catching his breath for a minute. All eyes were upon him with great anticipation.

Charles thought, *"Please, for Gods sake! Tell them to hurry up and release me."* The suspense was killing him.

Sir Andrew soon spoke. "Our most gracious Majesty has ordered that the lives of the young lads be spared." Thomas and Charles sighed with great relief. The Queen and Princess soon arrived, along with Lord Riley.

The Queen instructed her royal knights, "Untie the young lads at once." After Thomas and Charles were untied, they fell face first on the ground, bowing to the Queen in gratitude for her change of heart. The Queen ordered, "Young lads, arise," then walked over to Thomas, kissing him on both sides of his face. "I owe thee a debt of gratitude for saving the life of Princess Elizabeth."

Thomas replied as he bowed, "Your most gracious Majesty, truly it was a great honor."

The Queen turned her attention to Walter and Hubert in a normal tone of voice. "Because the Princess was not harmed, I shall show you two mercy."

The two sighed greatly relieved replying, "A thousand thanks, your most gracious Majesty."

The Queen pointed at them, changing her tone to an angry one, "By not torturing you to death! Quick! Off with their heads!" The royal guards quickly seized Walter and Hubert.

Sir Christopher pulled his sword out of its sheath as Princess Elizabeth screamed, "No! Do not!" Sir Christopher ignored the Princes, for nobody defies Bloody Mary and lives. He walked towards Hubert and Walter to chop off their heads.

Thomas quickly acted, dropping to the Queen's feet pleading. "Spare them for the sake of the debt of gratitude that you owe me!" Hearing this, Sir Christopher glanced at the Queen while he held his sword raised over the heads of Hubert and Walter.

The Queen raised her hand up, stopping. She looked down at Thomas and put her hand on his head. "Art thou certain? Shouldst thou instead ask of me great riches, it shall be granted."

Thomas remained bowing, but lifted his eyes up as he answered, "Yes, Your Most Gracious Majesty. Many thanks for repaying me with this favor." The Queen's pride stirred up inside. She contemplated the situation while she looked at Sir Christopher. The Queen was distressed with Thomas' request. However, she granted it with much respect.

The Queen turned her eyes toward Hubert and Walter. "Ye two are most fortunate, and along with the Princess, owe Thomas your lives."

The two bowed, trembling with fear, thanking the Queen. Then they thanked Thomas.

Princess Elizabeth bowed to the Queen saying, "Your Most Gracious Majesty, that which almost befell me 'tis no one's fault but mine own. Hubert and Walter are excellent swordsmen and fine guards. I do feel extremely safe, knowing they are here to protect me. Pray, could they remain my guards?"

The Queen contemplated for a minute before answering. "Thy request is granted. I do warrant that all the three of ye did learn a valuable lesson today."

The Princess embraced Queen Mary, saying, "Many thanks, good sister."

Afterwards, Princess Elizabeth walked over to Hubert and Walter, patting them on the backs, jokingly whispering, "Let us play hide and go seek."

Both guards shook their heads no as Hubert responded with an un-amused laugh, " Ha! Ha! Ha! No way!"

# CHAPTER XXVII
# BULLDOG, AT THE BALL.

The Queen instructed her helper, "Take Thomas and Charles in hand, and see to it that they are provided with proper attire, which they shall wear tonight for the royal banquet and ball at the castle." Hearing this, Thomas and Charles exchanged worried glances. The Queen noticed and asked, "What is troubling you young lads?"

Thomas replied, hesitantly, "With all due respect, Your Most Gracious Majesty, we have been away from our homes for quite some time now. Our parents must be very worried about us!"

The Queen raised her hand, saying, "Not to worry. Instruct one of my royal drivers how to get to your homes. Your parents shall be told your whereabouts and shall receive cordial invitations to attend the royal banquet and ball tonight. One of the royal carriages shall be provided to bring them here for the occasion, and to take them home again afterwards."

Both young lads bowed with appreciation as Charles replied, "God grant you mercy, Your Most Gracious Majesty."

Princess Elizabeth petted Moe as she looked at the Queen, "Can my pup's uncle attend the royal ball?"

No dog outside the royal family had ever attended such an event. The Queen pondered the question, while remembering an event in the past. The last royal event attended by a dog was the funeral of her father, Henry VIII. On that occasion, a lot of fluid from her father's body leaked out of the casket and spilled on the floor. One of the royal dogs licked Henry VIII up, causing shock and awe throughout the place. Any person in their right mind would say no to such a ludicrous request. As all know, Queen Mary was far from sane. She turned to Thomas, asking, "Will thy dog behave?"

Thomas answered, "Yes, Your Majesty."

The Queen rolled her eyes as she reluctantly complied, "Ah-so be it."

Princess Elizabeth smiled as she petted her pup, "Hear that, Little Moe?" Little Moe looked towards the Queen, wiggling her tail with a little thank you bark. "We get to meet your uncle tonight," the Princess said excitedly as she kissed her pup's head.

Thomas and Charles went with the Queen's helper, escorted by a few of the royal guards, to be fitted with proper clothing for the night's event. The Queen's helper picked out a magnificent black and purple outfit for Thomas and a magnificent turquoise and black outfit for Charles. Their new clothes were custom fitted in a timely manner. When the young lads arrived at the castle, the Princess, along with her cousins and friends, admired how handsome Thomas and Charles looked. The Princess told her friends, "I do declare, hands off the one in purple, for he is mine!" When Thomas' parents walked into the castle, Princess Elizabeth ran up to greet them, as Thomas introduced them to one another. The Princess had her pup in her arms and held him up to Dare. "Little Moe, this big dog is your uncle." As the Princess said this, Dare licked the pup's face. Afterwards, Dare licked the Princess' face as she petted him and said, "Dare is beautiful. He looks just like his brother, Terror."

Thomas restrained himself from rudely replying, "Ha, perhaps in looks and strength, tis all!" He managed to control his tongue and replied to the Princess with a slight touch of sarcasm, "God grant you mercy for that kind compliment." The Queen made Thomas and Charles, along with their families, guests of honor that night. They were invited to sit with the royal family for dinner. The Princess sat on Thomas' right, with her pup on the floor next to her, as Dare sat on his master's left side. People chuckled and smiled, seeing Dare's arms resting on the royal dinner table, looking like a distinguished young gentleman.

Princess Elizabeth said to Thomas' parents, "I am in great gratitude to your son, for he saved my life today."

Thomas's parents were shocked to hear this. "Zounds! How did this happen?" asked Thomas' father.

"Someone did try to abduct me. Shortly after my assailant grabbed me, your brave son did kill him, using a hammer to cave in his skull!" Immediately after this was said, Thomas cringed as his mother spit out her drink, choking.

"My son did what?" Thomas' surprised father responded as he attended to his wife.

The Queen interrupted, saying, "Master Thomas certainly did save Princess Elizabeth from her assailant, and after dinner he shall receive a nice surprise."

After the Queen said this, the Princess smiled at Thomas winking with a flirtatious smile as she rubbed his leg with her foot responding, "Most assuredly! Your son shall get a nice surprise." Thomas was taken by surprise to feel Princess Elizabeth's foot on his leg. He lunged forward, spilling some of his drink.

"Are you alright, Master Thomas?" Asked the Queen.

Thomas nodded his head yes, as the Princess replied, "I assure you, Master Thomas shall be quite fine." Charles saw the Princess give Thomas a foot massage and gave Thomas a smile with a nod. In fact, he himself was receiving a little massage under the table from Vadra. After the lovely dinner, they all danced. The Princess and Thomas danced as if they were floating on air. They made a striking looking couple.

After an hour of dancing, the Queen tapped the Princess on the shoulder. "May I cut in and dance with this fine lad?"

"Only if I get him back in one piece." answered Princess Elizabeth. Thomas gulped at the princess' comment. The Queen chuckled as she danced with him.

After that dance, the Queen stopped the musicians, and took Thomas' hand. She led him up to the center of the podium. "May I have your attention please for a moment. I have an announcement to make." The Queen paused. (At this time she was handed a royal gold medallion on a golden chain by one of her butlers.) "Earlier today, this fine young lad did risk his life to save my sister, Princess Elizabeth. Therefore, in recognition for his proven bravery and loyalty to the royal family, for which we are eternally grateful, I do present him with this royal gold medallion." (The Queen put the necklace over Thomas' neck as she said this.) "Outside the royal family, only eight other people have been presented these necklaces. Thomas is the ninth. This necklace is a sign of closeness to the royal family. It bears my insignia, that of Princess Elizabeth, and of our dearly, forever beloved father, King Henry VIII." (A sad look momentarily passed over the Queen's face when she mentioned her departed father.) "His mark was put on it just a few days prior to his departure from this world. This necklace shall allow Thomas and his friends to attend any royal event. It also allows Thomas entrance to the palace whenever he so desires."

Lord Riley was in the front of the podium with his nephew. With an absurd smile on his face, he was first to applaud. "Lucky son of a bitch" he whispered to his nephew, who stood there frowning with his arms crossed. "Do thou put your hands together, smile and clap for that bloody bastard!" Lord Riley mumbled, maintaining his smile without moving his lips. Vivian ignored this and kept his arms crossed. Lord Riley, noticing that people were looking at them strangely, gave Vivian a hard bump with his shoulder. "Do thou clap your hands, damn it! People are looking. Thou art an embarrassment." However, in truth, people were paying more attention to Lord Riley's absurd smile.

Vivian clapped but commented resentfully, "Your sword, uncle, is better than that necklace." At that moment the Queen was handed a sword, the sheath of which was covered with diamonds of three carats. The Queen pulled the sword out of its sheath and held it up to the crowd. They were awed by the shiny blade and impressive markings.

"I do also take pleasure in presenting Master Thomas with this rare sword, which bears on its blade the insignias of myself, of King Henry VIII, of King Henry VII, and of Princess Elizabeth." This sword was much more impressive than the sword that Lord Riley had been presented. He applauded as he turned glaring at his nephew, while wearing an even bigger absurd smile, he mumbled, "Hold thy bloody tongue, lest it be bloody, in fact." The Queen returned the sword to its sheath and handed it to Thomas, who received it with the utmost gratitude.

The Queen smiled at Thomas' reaction as she pulled her sword out, saying, "The title of master is no longer appropriate for thee. Kneel." Thomas did, humbly bowing. The Queen held the sword over Thomas' head. "By the power passed down to me by my father, King Henry VIII, I dub thee, Sir Thomas Avery Gentry. Moreover, thenceforth I declare this date to be known as "Sir Thomas Avery Gentry Day!" Dare, hearing his master's name mentioned, was the first to make noise by howling loudly. As he did, everyone at the party stood up and gave Sir Thomas a standing ovation. When the applause calmed down, the Queen took Sir Thomas' hand, and said, "Arise Sir Thomas Avery Gentry," and had him face the crowd.

Sir Thomas addressed the crowd, first with a soft stunned whistle, "Zounds, in me wildest dreams, never have I imagined a wonderful day like this to ever happen. 'Tis truly a great honor to be dub Sir Thomas by Your Most Gracious Majesty," (Sir Thomas said as he turned to her, bowing.) "My thanks. I do take great pride in me new title. As long as I live, I shall never bring shame to it."

The Queen hearing this smiled interrupting. "If thou dost, it shall be only once!"

The crowd laughed as the Princess shook her head, telling the Queen with her lips. "Stop that!"

Knowing that the Queen was serious, Sir Thomas covered his brief moment of fear with a smile, before addressing the crowd again. "The necklace and sword bestowed upon me are truly breathtaking! It has been a great privilege for me today making friends with Your Most Gracious Majesty and Princess Elizabeth. (Sir Thomas bowed to both the Queen and Princess as he mentioned them.) "'Twas a great honor to help save her life today. Although upon reflection, it seems that caving in the skull of Princess Elizabeth's attacker was also helping him, because knowing the amount of love our Majesty has for the Princess, I would hate to imagine what kind of torture she would have brought on Princess Elizabeth's assailant." The palace chuckled and agreed with this statement.

The Queen smiled commenting, "Sir Thomas speaks the truth!"

Well pleased, Sir Thomas looked at his sword and necklace. With a huge smile, he said, "Many good thanks for these wonderful gifts, Your Most

Gracious Majesty; receiving them is truly a great honor. I shall cherish them all the days of my life, and shall wear my medallion with great pride."

Pleased with Sir Thomas' reaction, the Queen smiled, and nodded her head in his direction.

Sir Thomas bowed as he kissed the Queen's hand, then raised it, shouting, "Long live the Queen!" The whole palace immediately followed echoing, "Long live the Queen." When Sir Thomas stepped off of the podium, he received hugs, kisses and congratulations from just about everyone. Even Lord Riley attempted to give him a hug, a phony one of course. But as he approached with open arms, Dare snarled, exposing his fangs. Needless to say, Lord Riley immediately backed away.

When Sir Thomas had been thoroughly congratulated, Princess Elizabeth approached Sir Thomas and Queen Mary with Moe in her arms, asking, "Pray, might I be excused, along with Sir Thomas, Charles, and my cousin, so we can go to my room and play with my pup?"

Dare, as always, was close to his master's side. Seeing this, the Queen answered, "Thou mayest, if thou dost behave and dost take Dare with thee."

Princess Elizabeth, exhaling hard, whispered, "Damn!" She did not want Dare in her room with them. However, she answered bowing, though with a phony smile, "Of course. My thanks, Your Most Gracious Majesty."

# CHAPTER XXVIII
# TORN HEART

Upon entering her room, Princess Elizabeth put her pup on the bed and then walked outside on her window balcony with her cousin. "Do come," she called to Sir Thomas and Charles, "I do wish ye both to see the beautiful view from my balcony."

As Charles approached the window, his eyes looked up and down lustfully at Vadra. "'Twould be impossible for the beautiful view outside your window to compare to the beautiful view I now behold!" Vadra blushed, hearing Charles' comment, as he took her hand and kissed it.

Sir Thomas walked up to Princess Elizabeth and looked all around from her balcony. "Zounds! 'Tis truly the most beautiful view ever I have seen." Princess Elizabeth looked at Charles and her cousin, who were engaged in a kiss. Charles didn't even glance at the beautiful view. His eyes were either closed or on Vadra. The Princess turned her head sideways, putting her face close to Sir Thomas' lips. Sir Thomas inhaled the Princess' perfume. "My Princess, you certainly do smell good." Princess Elizabeth interpreted that as a sign of interest. She wrapped her arms around his hips and kissed him on the lips. Sir Thomas' hands shook a little as he slowly wrapped his arms around her and returned her kiss. Dare knew that his master felt uncomfortable because he was in love with Emily. Therefore, Dare barked, startling everyone and causing all to jump.

With a touch of anger in her tone, the Princess said, "Do shut thy mouth, thou dumb dog!" Because of her comment, Sir Thomas had a hurt look on his face. Princess Elizabeth knew that her words had hurt his feelings. She took his hand and said, "Pray forgive me, for I did not mean that."

Looking down, Sir Thomas took the Princess' other hand. "There is no need to apologize to me. It is Charles and I who need to apologize."

Princess Elizabeth was surprised to hear this. She pulled her hands away. "I do not understand. What need is there for the two of ye to apologize?"

Hearing this, Vadra stopped kissing Charles, who brushed his face off and asked, "Yes, indeed. What need is there for thee to apologize?" Charles stood there, baffled. His mouth was open as he tried to answer, but was unable to say a word.

All the confused eyes turned to Sir Thomas as he answered Princess Elizabeth's question. "I have pledged loyalty to another beautiful lady, and the same is true of me good friend Charles. It would not be proper for either of us to betray our ladies and lead you on."

"Is this true Charles?" Vadra asked with a very perturbed expression. "Art thou planning to lead me on?" Charles remained speechless with his mouth open, shocked Sir Thomas had even mentioned their lady loves. "Well, if that be the case," Vadra said as she slapped Charles across the face and pointed to the door, "do thou take your leave!" As Charles walked towards the door, he hit his hand against his knuckles giving both Sir Thomas and Dare a couple of mean looks. Vadra started complaining bitterly as she turned towards the Princess. "Can you. . . !" The Princess held her hand up, interrupting.

"Pray, leave us! We shall be out shortly." Vadra took a deep frustrating breath as she walked out the door. Sir Thomas sat on the Princess bed, his head held down in shame as he petted Moe with one hand and Dare with the other. Princess Elizabeth put one hand on Sir Thomas' head, running her fingers through his long brunette hair. "I do believe that congratulations are in order for the noble and handsome Sir Thomas."

"I beg your pardon?" Sir Thomas asked, surprised.

"For being the first to break the heart of a Princess." Sir Thomas gently took the Princess' hand, kissing it as bowed and knelt.

"Pray, forgive me, my Princess. I am in great distress, knowing that I have hurt you." Princess Elizabeth put her index finger on his chin, and raised it so their eyes could meet.

"Pray, tell me Sir Thomas, doth the lady who does hold the key to your heart, have eyes and beauty that compare to that of a Princess'?" Sir Thomas was in a bad dilemma. If he answered yes, the Princess would have her heart hurt even more. If he answered no, the Princess would probably reply, "Then do shut thy mouth and kiss me, and do not fret over your former lady-love!"

Sir Thomas cleverly answered, "My lady's beauty and my Princess' beauty are equally second to none. However, with all due respect, my Princess, I have known my lady for quite some time and have more of a connection with her."

Hearing this, the Princess turned and walked outside on her balcony window and shed a tear. "Never have I heard of anyone who could win the heart of a man over a Princess."

Sir Thomas followed, putting his hands gently on her shoulders, "Make no mistake my Princess! I do love you and have proven I will kill for you! If need be, I would also die for you!"

Princess Elizabeth wiped a few more tears from her eyes and turned to him. "Ha, 'tis a good thing for thee that I do not have my sister's or father's temper, at least yet, for that would have been the case." After saying this she hugged Sir Thomas, shedding more tears on his handsome purple shirt. Princess Elizabeth soon pulled away. She looked up, staring in his eyes with the bright full moon in the background. "Although I have only known thee for one day, thou art my first love. My heart doth break at not being kissed and embraced in thine arms. If I cannot have this, 'tis best that after tonight we do not see each other again." Sir Thomas turned sideways, putting his hands on the Princess' balcony rail as he stared at the bright stars. An uncomfortable silence passed before Sir Thomas replied, "I am so sorry my Princess. I cannot give you that"

Disappointed, Princess Elizabeth turned and walked back into her bedroom and over to her pup, and as she picked him up, she sarcastically whispered looking at Dare. "My thanks, thou crazy beast! Couldst thou not have stayed at home?" Dare looked at the Princess surprised, with his head turned sideways as if to say. "What did I do?" Princess Elizabeth dried her tears and put on a phony smile saying, "We had better leave now; people are waiting for us." They walked outside Princess Elizabeth's door. Vadra was outside with arms crossed and nose in the air, looking away from Charles who stood there speechless, thinking, *"Why could Thomas not keep his big mouth shut?"*

Princess Elizabeth told Sir Thomas, "Ye three go back to the party. We shall be there shortly."

As Charles walked back to the party, he looked at Sir Thomas and Dare and shook his head saying, "I am too irate to talk about this right now!"

Vadra sniffled to the Princess, "How can those two buffoons possibly think about other ladies when they are in our presence? Why, they are not even in the same class as we are." Vadra paused with a sigh, "And to think that they are worried about hurting our feelings! We are the ones who would have shattered their hearts, just as we have done to several other young gentlemen in the past!"

Tears from the eyes of Princess Elizabeth began dripping onto the floor. "I do need to be alone right now," said Princess Elizabeth, as she ran back into her room with her pup in her arms, closing and locking the door.

"This can not be happening!" Vadra said, shaking her head, "Beautiful Princesses never have their hearts broken." Vadra rested her head on Princess Elizabeth's door. She raised her hand to knock, but heard the Princess cry like a baby. Vadra left, baffled. Sir Thomas returned for the remainder of the ball, feeling depressed. He kept quiet, shaking hands with the people who congratulated him.

When Sir Thomas and his family left the castle, the Queen walked them out saying. "I do wonder where Princess Elizabeth might be. 'Tis rather rude of her not say goodbye."

Vadra walked out with them. Slowly her narrowed, angry eyes shifted from Charles to Sir Thomas as she answered the Queen. "I do regret to inform your grace that the Princess is not feeling well."

"Oh! What is the matter?" the Queen asked, concerned.

Vadra sighed dramatically before answering, "She doth have a pain in her heart."

The Queen turned abruptly, "Heavens! That could be fatal. I had best check on her."

Vadra's angry eyes remained on Sir Thomas as she spoke quietly to him so the Queen couldn't overhear. "It certainly can be fatal . . . for the person who caused it!" Sir Thomas gulped with fear.

As the Queen went running into the entrance of the castle, Princess Elizabeth came out. "Art thou alright, my child?" The Queen asked deeply concerned.

"Yes, I am quite fine." The Princess answered, glaring at her cousin, and knowing that Vadra had opened her big fat mouth. "By your leave, I would like to thank my hero alone."

Queen Mary nodded her head once as she answered, "Yes, my child. But do take Sir Thomas' powerful dog with thee for protection."

The Princess thanked the Queen, then walked with Sir Thomas and Dare alone saying, "I shall not allow my pride to prevent me from departing on a good note from the one who saved my life, for which action I am eternally grateful. One day when I am upon the throne, thou shalt be properly rewarded with great riches."

Sir Thomas answered as he took the Princess' hand, "Your safety is my reward."

The two continued to walk, and looking down, Princess Elizabeth continued, "The words that I said to thee earlier were very arrogant. My conduct was unbecoming a Princess."

Sir Thomas raised Princess Elizabeth's hand up to his lips and kissed it. "You did nothing wrong, my Princess. You did not know there was someone in my life for whom I had strong feelings."

The Princess suddenly stopped and looked at him. Her eyes reflected the beauty of the stars that were seen for millions of miles away that night. "I do not wish for thee to answer me; just listen. Today is a day that I shall remember for the rest of my life. My heart shall never forget thee. If things do not work out with your lady, come to me and give us a chance." Sir Thomas put his hands on Princess Elizabeth's shoulder, kissing her forehead.

"I shall never forget you either, my Princess."

Princess Elizabeth responded, timidly staring in his eyes, "If the young Sir wills, let me feel thy embrace and lips pressed against mine with no

hesitation, just one time before thou goest. No one else will have to know."
Sir Thomas granted the Princess' wish. He kissed and embraced the Princess
with no hesitation for a long time. Dare sat next to them with his head turned
sideways, watching without interfering, that is until the Queen came close by
with her guards to check on the Princess. That's when he barked. Sir Thomas
suddenly stopped and looked in the direction where Dare was barking. Two
seconds latter, the Queen was seen.

"There ye two are," said the Queen smiling, "I was starting to get worried
about ye."

Princess Elizabeth, upset at being disturbed, responded harshly, "We are
quite fine, thank you!"

The Queen cringed a little, knowing that the Princess was upset with her.
She turned to Sir Thomas and said, "Thy parents and family are waiting for
thee in the royal carriage."

Even more upset and rolling her eyes, Princess Elizabeth responded,
"Alright! We shall be there shortly!"

The Queen turned around abruptly. "Alright, I shall leave the two of thee
alone now. Be not long."

Princess Elizabeth shook her head, still upset that they had been interrupted.
She gave Sir Thomas a quick kiss on his lips before saying," I do think we
had best return now and say our goodbyes." After saying his goodbyes, Sir
Thomas hopped into the royal carriage with a huge smile on his face, which
remained there all the way home, while the frowning Charles keeping his
arms folded, glared at Thomas and Dare all the way. Early the next morning,
Charles knocked on Sir Thomas' door to give him a piece of his mind.

Sir Thomas answered the door and said "Hello," but before he could say
another word, Charles commenced complaining bitterly.

"I do have many a thing to say to thee, so thou wilt keep thy mouth shut
and listen! First of all, thou are an idiot! Princess Elizabeth is beautiful. How
could thou have not returned her kiss, as I did Vadra's? By rejecting her and
saying that thou art spoken for, thou couldst well have caused us both to have
our heads chopped off! And why needst thou to involve me? I was having
a good time with Vadra!" Sir Thomas had his finger over his lips and was
pointing behind him with his thumb, in an attempt to signal that Emily and
Sara were directly behind him, listening to every word. Charles refused to
pay attention and continued his lament. "How couldst thou have the audacity
to tell those two beautiful ladies that we were with last night that thou didst
not wish to hurt their feelings, for we are not even in the same class as they
are! They probably have a dozen young gentleman friends and just wanted
to act out their lusty desires with us!" Sir Thomas kept pointing inside and

behind him, holding a finger to his lips, desperately trying to silence Charles, who kept rambling. "Do thou not silence me! I am going to speak and thou art going to listen! After all, last night thou hast ruined what could have been the best night of me life!"

Suddenly Sir Thomas' door swung open. Sara, in a serious fit of rage, ran in front of Charles and slapped his face. "So, in other words, I am not in the same class as this tramp Vadra, whose company thou dost prefer to mine own."

"No! No! Give me leave to explain!" Charles said, trotting backwards, blocking some of Sara's slaps that were going near his face as she continued complaining.

"Now thou shalt be the one who to shut up whilst I speak!" As Charles was experiencing Sara's wrath, Emily slowly approached Sir Thomas in a very alluring manner.

When he tried to speak, she put her finger over her lips, "Shhh." Emily didn't say a word. She wrapped her arms around Sir Thomas, tackling him to the ground while she lay on top, kissing him. Weeks later, Sara and Charles eventually made up, thanks to countless amount of hours of bowing, scraping, toadying and rump kissing by Charles.

# CHAPTER XXIX
# WOOING STRICTLY FORBIDDEN

A few months later, Terror had fully recovered. Lord Riley, seeing him well and able to seize cattle and bring them to the ground again with ease, announced another fight to the death, this time between Terror and Brahma the Bull. However, the puppies that Terror had produced before his last fight with Enormous Elias did not turn out as Lord Riley was hoping as they grew. They were good fighting dogs, but none of them were as good as Terror. No matter how much Lord Riley inbred them, he just couldn't produce another Terror. Lord Riley's favorite female Emerald was in heat again. The last time this happened, he had inbred Terror to his mother. This produced eight dogs that were terrible specimens which Lord Riley killed. Two dogs turned out to be fine fighting dogs, but still were nothing like Terror. So Lord Riley thought of a fiendish plan to steel Blaze from Robert and breed Blaze to Emerald in hopes of producing more killer fighting dogs like Terror and Dare. Lord Riley waited until Sunday. He learned from staking out Robert's house that every Sunday morning, Robert attended Church. So after Robert had left for church, Lord Riley threw a few small stones in Robert's yard near Blaze, to get his attention. Sly Ann heard the rocks also and got an eerie feeling about this.

She looked at Blaze, barking as if to say, "Do not go outside our yard! I think there is great danger for you out there." Blaze knew what Sly Ann was trying to tell him, so he cautiously crawled underneath the fence, sniffing and looking around. A fish soon caught his attention. Blaze cautiously walked towards the fish as Sly Ann continued to warn. When Blaze came near, Lord Riley pulled on a rope, causing a large net to drop down from the trees. Blaze tried to jump clear of the trap. He almost made it, but was a fraction of a second too late. Blaze squirmed, desperately trying to free himself from the net. He was seconds away from succeeding when Lord Riley quickly ran out from behind the bushes where he was hiding and wrapped Blaze up securely in the net. Blaze was unable to escape.

Lord Riley carried Blaze a little ways away to the place where he had left his carriage, and carefully put Blaze in it. Smilingly Lord Riley said as he whipped the reins riding off to his estate. "Stop squirming and conserve thy strength, for thou shalt have need of it to woo my favorite bitch." Sly Ann crawled underneath the fence, chasing Lord Riley's carriage a little ways before realizing that she had better wait until her master came home.

After church, when Robert approached his home, he heard Sly Ann barking sadly. He knew something was definitely wrong. He ran to the fence where Sly Ann was, asking, "What is wrong?" Robert looked around his yard. All the dogs were there except for Blaze. Robert turned to Sly Ann, asking "Canst thou take me to where Blaze is?"

Sly Ann immediately crawled underneath the fence, looking at her master and giving a bark as if to say, "Follow me." Robert followed and Sly Ann took him to the place where Blaze had been captured. Robert looked around. He found the rope that Lord Riley had used to help capture Blaze. Robert also found pieces of net used in capturing Blaze. The first thing that popped in his mind was Lord Riley's phony, lying, smiling face.

Out of rage Robert kicked a rock yelling, "Damn you, Lord Riley!" Sly Ann had led him to where Lord Riley had entered his carriage. Robert crouched down and saw wheel tracks there. He patted Sly Ann on the head, saying "Good dog!" The two followed the wheel tracks as Robert told Sly Ann, "That bloody bastard's beating shall be legendary." The tracks went near his brother's house. At the time, Sir Thomas and Dare happened to be outside pulling weeds together. When Robert and Sly Ann approached, Dare took off running to greet them. Sir Thomas followed close behind. Dare soon caught up with Robert, knocking him to the ground and trying to play wrestle with him. Robert was not in the mood. He tried throwing Dare off while yelling obscenities at him. Dare knew that something was greatly disturbing Robert, so he immediately got off.

Sir Thomas saw and heard what was going on from a short distance away. He ran over concerned. This was the first time he had ever heard his uncle Robert swear. Sir Thomas asked, "What is wrong, uncle?"

As he rose to his feet, wiping off the saliva from Dare's tongue, Thomas' uncle replied. "Do tell thy damn dog never to do that again!" Sir Thomas stood there speechless as his uncle took several deep breaths, before realizing that Dare and his nephew had done nothing wrong. They were just taking the brunt of his frustrations. So in a changed tone of voice he said, "I do love both of thee very much and am sorry. 'Tis merely that right now I truly do need to be alone with Sly Ann. Pray, leave us. We shall join the two of thee very soon." After saying this, Robert and Sly Ann continued to follow the carriage tracks. Sir Thomas and Dare exchanged baffled looks, both knowing that something was definitely wrong.

Sir Thomas petted Dare's shoulder, telling him, "Well, thou dost know what to do. I do wish that I could follow along, but if I did so, 'twould make too much noise. Mine uncle would then know that I do spy upon him, but he will not know that thou art doing so." Sir Thomas got down on one knee, patting his dog's head as Dare licked him. "Do thou be careful, my friend, and do take care of my favorite uncle." With that Dare turned running to catch up with Robert. Sir Thomas went to his uncle's house to wait. When Sir Thomas arrived, he looked around and noticed that Blaze was not there. Sir Thomas put two and two together. It didn't take long for him to realize that Lord Riley had stolen Blaze in an attempt to create another Terror or Dare. Besides, Lord Riley's estate was in the direction his uncle was walking. Sir Thomas left, running towards Lord Riley's.

Robert constantly looked over his shoulder and all around, trying to make sure that his nephew wasn't following. Robert knew that there was a good chance of some violence. He didn't want his nephew exposed to any of it or to get hurt. But no matter how hard he looked he could not see Dare, who quietly followed and kept himself hidden in bushes. When Robert and Sly Ann eventually arrived at Lord Riley's, they heard him in the back yard. Robert peeked through a fence. What he saw infuriated him even more.

Without scruples, Lord Riley threw Blaze on top of Emerald, ordering them to "Make me some bloody killers, bitch!"

Robert shouted at the top of his lungs, "You bloody bastard! Did I not forbid you to use my dog for wooing? I do demand that Blaze be returned to me immediately!" Lord Riley, seeing only Robert and Sly Ann, gave a sinister chuckle as he let Terror out of his cage. The two slowly and arrogantly approached Robert and Sly Ann. Seeing this, Dare crept closer, quiet as a cat, keeping hidden behind bushes, and watching cautiously.

Lord Riley came within inches of Robert's face and threatened him in a sarcastic and fighting tone. "I am not using your dog! Why, I am using my dog. I do suggest most strongly that you vacate my premises at once!" Robert, being a strong God-fearing believer, tried to control his anger, but even he couldn't so. His body shook all over from being in a state of rage. Lord Riley, seeing that Robert was not budging, told him, "So be it," then took a swing at Robert with his right hand. Robert blocked the punch with his left arm while at the same time grabbing Lord Riley on the throat with his right hand.

While pulling Lord Riley's face close to his own, Robert screamed, "You piece of filth! Listen to me! If ever you try to steal any more of my dogs, I do promise you shall wish that you had never been born." Hearing his master in a state of rage, Blaze quickly finished wooing Emerald, jumped off her back, leaped over Lord Riley's high fence and stood by his master's side. At that moment, Sly Ann was having a face off with Terror, who would not attack because he was recently trained not to do so under any circumstances unless given the verbal command by his master. Terror was afraid that if he attacked, he would get hit with a whip. This is why Terror didn't defend his master and remained still, because Lord Riley was unable to command.

Robert, seeing Blaze by his side safe out of Lord Riley's yard, thought, *"Good, now we can leave."* Robert lifted Lord Riley up with both hands on the throat, throwing him about eight feet into the air and causing him to land flat on his back. Lord Riley lay there with the wind knocked out of him, gasping for air. Robert looked at Terror, who was foaming at the mouth. Terror was crouched back eagerly waiting to attack, thinking, "At any moment now I should hear the attack command from my master. When I do, I shall rip these dogs and this man to shreds." Dare remained hidden, knowing that if his presence were known, it would only make matters worse. From a short distance away, he watched intensely what was going on, slowly and quietly creeping closer and closer from behind the bushes, trying to get in a good position from which he could make a good surprise attack on Terror, if he were to attack.

# CHAPTER XXX
# BROTHER VERSES BROTHER FOR
# NO PROFIT OF ANOTHER

Terror stared into Robert's eyes. Robert felt Terror's evil stare, knowing that the worst thing he could do would be to stare back. This would be saying in dog language, "I accept your challenge." Therefore, Robert very intelligently looked away and watched Terror out of the corner of his eye while slowly walking backwards with his two dogs, knowing full well that Terror could easily tear his dogs apart. Robert also knew that they had to get out of there before Lord Riley was able to speak and give Terror the attack command. Once Robert and his dogs backed about thirty feet away from Lord Riley, Terror turned, looking back at his master, and started to walk toward Robert. Seeing this, Robert knew that this was their opportunity to run for their lives. As soon as they did so, Lord Riley cleared his throat.

Pointing at Robert, Lord Riley yelled in a raspy tone, "Kill, Terror! Kill!" Terror took off after Robert, moving three times faster than Robert could run. Seeing Terror committing to attack, Dare knew that he had to intervene to save Robert's life. He came out from behind the bushes where he was hiding, running so fast that no one saw him coming. When Terror approached a distance of six feet in back of Robert, he jumped, and so did Dare, also six feet away on Robert's right side. Robert looked back and saw Terror, with his eyes crazed and mouth wide open, flying in the air at him. Robert's eyes bulged with fear, seeing humongous fangs speedily heading straight for his face. Terror's fangs were two inches away when Dare intercepted him. His front paws collided with Terror's back right leg, knocking him to the ground. Both dogs quickly sprung back to their feet, circling around one another, snarling with huge fangs fully exposed. Seeing this, Lord Riley commented, "Damn! I am about to see the best dog fight in history and will not make a penny off of it."

Robert turned to Sly Ann and Blaze. "Ye two sit and stay! Do not try to help your friend. He is better off on his own. Ye two would just get killed in vain." Blaze and Sly Ann were trained exceptionally well. They remained sitting, barking the whole time, reluctantly obeying their master.

At that moment, Vivian showed up on his horse, and his eyes lit up intensely. "Alas," he told his uncle, "Our dog is about to fight Dare to the death and will probably win! I must get to my father and inform him, along with my friends, to come over and witness this." Vivian rode his fastest towards home. On his way, he passed by Henry's house, who happened to be outside with Francis and Stanley, throwing rocks at bottles. Vivian rode by shouting, "Go over to Lord Riley's. Terror and Dare are fighting there!" The three dropped their rocks at once, without saying a word, and ran their fastest over to Lord Riley's. Vivian soon arrived home. "Father! Father!" he shouted. "Come quickly, Terror is fighting Dare right now at Uncle's!" Vivian then turned his horse around, and headed back to his uncle's estate. His father threw the book he was reading into the air and jumped on his horse, following close behind Vivian.

As Vivian, his father, and his acquaintances were on their way, the two dogs engaged in fighting. They leaped into the air at each other, knocking one another to the ground. Robert knew that these two dogs were equally matched and that either dog could win. He also knew that both dogs had a strong chance of dying if this fight wasn't soon stopped. Robert yelled at Lord Riley, "Call your dog off at once!"

Lord Riley ignored Robert. Lord Riley desperately wanted to have a couple more dogs like Terror and Dare. If he called Terror off, Robert would take Blaze home. Lord Riley then wouldn't be able to try breeding Blaze again with Emerald. Lord Riley was also extremely entertained by the fight. He shook his head at Robert's command replying, "Nay, call yours off first!" Robert wasn't naïve. He knew that if he did so, Lord Riley still wouldn't call off Terror. This would give Terror an advantage because Dare would be distracted.

The dogs fought evenly over the next several minutes, each getting little bites in, and each desperately trying to get hold of the other's throat first. Robert chased Lord Riley and soon caught him. Holding Lord Riley in a tight headlock, Robert demanded, "Call Terror off at once!"

With tears coming down his face from being choked, Lord Riley looked towards the dogs. He didn't see or hear them fighting any more. He only saw a cloud of dust. When the dust cleared, Lord Riley had an upset and defeated expression on his face, not from being choked until he was red in the face, but because Terror also was in a submissive hold, pinned to the ground by his neck. Dare stood directly on top of his brother, with his jaws firmly wrapped around his brother's throat.

Francis, Henry, and Stanley showed up at that moment. Seeing that Dare had a submissive hold on Terror, they glanced at one another fearfully. "Oh, no! Not again," Henry said, as they turned and ran inside Lord Riley's manor where they would be safe from Dare. Cautiously they watched from the window.

Dare knew that Terror was his brother. At that moment, Dare could have very easily killed Terror, but he didn't want to do so. As Dare held his brother, he remembered when they were little puppies playing with each other, loving one another; and he remembered how sad he and his littermates were when Lord Riley took their brother away from them. Lord Riley had successfully turned a dog with an outstanding temperament into a heartless killer. Knowing this broke Dare's heart. Dare also distinctly remembered how his brother had saved his life when they were puppies. He held Terror, trying to tell him by crying softly, "Brother I love you. Please do not make me kill you." Terror felt his brother's mercy bite, and he knew Dare wanted to spare his life. At that moment, a little tear from Dare's eye trickled down Terror's face; this drop was water to the seeds of love Thomas had planted. However, Terror's heart was still burdened with rage and hate. Terror tried to shake himself free so he could kill his brother, but the more he tried, the more pain he felt from Dare's powerful jaws.

Seeing that Dare had won, Lord Riley surrendered. "Terror, stop fighting. Come here!" Lord Riley paused, straining for breath. "Robert, I have submitted to your demands. Now you do likewise. Call Dare off and release me."

Seeing that Dare had a submissive hold on Terror, Robert replied, "Not on your life! I am not gullible. If I call Dare off, how do I know that you will not command Terror to attack again?"

Lord Riley was released from his headlock. He tried to get the kinks out by moving his neck around as he answered, "Because I give me word."

Robert chuckled before responding, "Your word means absolutely nothing."

Terror suddenly came up with a plan. He felt his brother's love and mercy, and used it against his brother by acting as if he were choking and unconscious. Noticing his brother was no longer squirming or growling, Dare thought his brother was badly injured. Therefore, Dare let go of Terror's throat and turned to go check on Robert and his dogs to make sure they were all right. "Good dog Dare. I am proud of thee. Let us go home now." Right after Robert said this, Terror rose up foaming at the mouth, his fangs fully exposed. Dare and Robert had their backs turned to him. Terror was even more determined to kill his brother, now more than ever.

Seeing this, Lord Riley sucker punched Robert in the stomach, causing him to bend over, and then tackled him to the ground. Meanwhile, Terror lunged at Dare, and the two fought again as Lord Riley and Robert wrestled. Robert soon had Lord Riley in a headlock again. As soon as he did, Vivian and his father arrived.

Jumping off his horse, Vivian screamed with great excitement, "Kill, Terror! Kill!" as his father jumped off his horse and kicked Robert in the face, freeing Lord Riley from Robert's grasp. Robert put up a good fight but was outnumbered and ended up in a submission hold. Both Lord Riley and Sherman III pushed Robert's face into the mud, while another cloud of dust formed from the dogfight. All eyes watched intently as the dust slowly cleared. Lord Riley and Sherman III were ready to release Robert and run for their lives if they saw Dare the victor again. But this time, Dare was the one in a submissive hold. Terror stood on top of him with his jaws wrapped around Dare's throat. Terror was victorious. Laughing, Lord Riley and Sherman III kept Robert pinned. Vivian ran around, jumping up and down, and joyfully shouting, celebrating sweet victory while pointing his finger at Henry, Stanley and Francis, "Yes! Did I not tell ye that Terror would defeat Dare! Come out of my uncle's manor, ye cowards! My family always has owned and always shall own the best fighting dogs in the world." With raised hands, Vivian praised Terror. "Behold the legendary Terror! What beast can withstand such fierce jaws?" Vivian continued to shout for joy for several more minutes before he eventually calmed down and lowered his hands. He took several deep breaths as he looked at Dare, who lay helplessly pinned to the ground, begging for mercy with his eyes. Vivian, feeling the need for revenge, mocked him, saying, "Foolish dog! Thou shouldst never have come over here, for thou art now about to be chewed up into little pieces, just as I predicted would happen if thou didst fight Terror!" A vindictive smile filled Vivian's face while he told Terror, "Go ahead! Bite his head off and indulge yourself with his bloody guts!"

Lord Riley rubbed Robert's face in the mud with his foot, as he also mocked. "I warned you to get off of my property! When Terror is finished biting Dare's head off, he shall come over here and do likewise to you." Lord Riley then turned towards the dogs. "Enough with the foreplay, Terror k-," Lord Riley that moment was abruptly interrupted from saying the word *kill* by Sir Thomas, who had just arrived. Lord Riley held his tongue for a moment, chuckling. Sir Thomas ran over to the dogs, screaming, "No, Terror. Grant mercy to thy brother!" Robert screamed at his nephew, with great fear for his nephew's life. "Sir Thomas, I do order thee to run away from here." But Sir Thomas did not heed his uncle's order.

Lord Riley shook his head as he looked at Sir Thomas. "Foolish lad! I have completely broken Terror. You would be better off right now if you were in front of a hungry Lion!" Lord Riley and Sherman III watched chuckling all the more.

"What a fool the lad is." Sherman III commented, shaking his head.

Lord Riley bent down and whispered in Robert's ear, while rubbing his face in the mud some more with his foot, "Yes indeed, my cousin is correct. Your nephew is a fool, and because of it, he shall also die!"

Robert squirmed so his head was away from the mud momentarily. Glaring at Lord Riley, he yelled, "I do warn you, do not lay hand on my nephew!"

Chuckling, Lord Riley replied, "Or what?" as he pushed Robert's face back into the mud again, silencing him. "I certainly have enjoyed these extended preliminaries, although it is time now for ye fools to die!" Lord Riley paused and clasped his hands together, making a clapping sound, before giving the command, "Terror, kill!" Oddly, Terror did not respond. He kept his eye on Sir Thomas, remembering the kindness and love Sir Thomas had shown when he had healed him. The seeds of love that Sir Thomas had planted in Terror's heart now received water and soil from Dare's cry's and loving mercy grip. At that moment, Terror's seeds of love started springing forth in his heart and became manifested. His mean snarl and evil eyes full of rage and hate began to transform into eyes of great sorrow and affection for his brother and Sir Thomas. Terror's mean snarl was slowly replaced with a cute, droopy, wrinkled face. Ever since Terror had been taken away from his littermates, he had never felt any love, except recently from Sir Thomas and Dare. Even when Terror would win a fight, Lord Riley never showed him any affection.

Lord Riley continued to order Terror to kill, becoming angrier and angrier each time, as Sir Thomas kept pleading, "Pray, Terror! Show mercy on me best friend, your brother. Do thou release him and be my dog too! I promise, thou shalt be loved for the rest of your life, which will be most unlike your life with this evil Lord!"

Lord Riley became infuriated, seeing Terror's strange transformation and watching him disobey a direct order. His jaw dropped in disbelief as he said, shaking his head, "This can not be happening." Furiously he ran to the side of his manor, yelling as he grabbed his whip, "Terror, I said kill!" Just as Lord Riley grabbed his whip, Terror released Dare. All eyes looked in shock at what just happened, while Sir Thomas ran over to Dare, wrapping his arms around him while patting Terror on the head. On the other hand, Lord Riley shook his head in utter disgust. "This is me worst nightmare: the best fighting dog in the world showing mercy. That shall be changed." Furious at Terror, Lord Riley threw his whip back, and began to whip him hard.

Sir Thomas reacted by screaming, "No!" and leaping in front of Terror.

Sir Thomas wasn't as big as Terror, so could not shield and protect him. Lord Riley went to whip Terror again. Terror cried out, knowing that the only way his master would stop would be if he fought his brother to the death, which he was not going to do. Therefore, Terror humbly lay motionless, crying in pain and prepared to be whipped to death. Dare, on the other hand, never had a bond with Lord Riley. He was not about to just lie there and let some demented person swing a whip near his master, striking his brother. So the next time Lord Riley snapped his whip at Terror, Dare jumped eight feet high, and intercepted it with his mouth. When Dare landed on the ground, he jerked the whip violently back with his neck. This caused Lord Riley to fall in the mud face first. While snarling, Dare slowly turned his head sideways toward Sherman III, who still had Robert in a submissive hold. Sherman III, seeing Dare's furious eyes staring in his own, instantly released Robert, and dashed into Lord Riley's manor, followed closely by his son, where they joined Henry, Francis and Stanley. Meanwhile, Dare's furious eyes moved to Lord Riley, who had just cleared the mud from his eyes. A second later Dare chased him and soon caught him by the back of the skull. Dare ripped a chunk of hair off Lord Riley's head while pulling him to the ground, forcing him to land on his back. Dare then wrapped his jaws around Lord Riley's neck. He was moments away from crushing Lord Riley's neck and removing it from his body, but was distracted by Terror, who barked loudly, stopping him.

"Let him go!" Terror strongly communicated through his barks. "Even though he was abusive towards me, he was my master and fed me. I still have feelings towards him."

Dare reluctantly respected his brother's request, letting go of Lord Riley, and backed away. His fangs were fully exposed as he stared deep into Lord Riley's eyes with an angry growl as if to say, "You have no idea how lucky you are and how much restraint I am using right now to not tear you apart." This time when Lord Riley made a mess in his pants, it wasn't liquid.

Dare and Sir Thomas ran over to Robert to help him up. Sir Thomas took off his shirt to wipe his uncle's bloody lip and to clean the mud off of his face. His uncle was a little beaten up but was basically fine. They then walked away from there. Terror stayed behind. Sir Thomas called out to him, "Come with us. Thou art now part of our family."

Terror followed as Lord Riley warned, "Terror is my dog! 'Tis against the law to steal him. If you do, I shall report you to the proper authorities."

Robert warned in return, "Terror is his own dog! He doth walk away from you of his own free will, unlike when you stole Blaze from me. Therefore do shut your mouth, lest I allow Dare to do what he wills with you!" Hearing this, Lord Riley became quiet as Robert and his family continued on their way home. When they arrived at home, Terror and Dare played chase and wrestled with each other just like when they were little puppies. When they were finished playing, Robert looked sadly at Terror as he petted him with compassion. He knew Terror was an abused dog, used against his will to fight in the pit. Robert got a towel and cleaned up Terror's neck where Dare had him pinned in the fight. Sir Thomas did likewise to Dare. Robert then got some food for both of them to eat. After eating, Terror sat in front of Sir Thomas, wiggling his tail staring deep into his eyes, and telling him telepathically, "Please mean what you said about letting me be your dog. I will be a good dog, I promise. Please do not send me back to my cruel master. I do not want to kill for his pleasure any more, nor live that kind of life. All I want is to love and be loved as my brother is."

Sir Thomas, seeing this in Terror's eyes, hugged him and said, "Do not dread, my big friend. I will not allow any more harm come to thee." Sir Thomas turned his eyes upward and looked sadly at his uncle. "Do you really believe Lord Riley will call the authorities on us?"

His uncle, with his head down, answered, "Yes, I do."

Sir Thomas gave a quick movement of his head as he replied, "Damn it!" Then he paused a second, taking a deep breath, "We must help Terror, but how?"

Robert walked over to his nephew. Getting down on one knee and putting his left hand on his nephew's shoulder, he answered, while petting Terror. "Unfortunately it is starting to get dark, so I can not leave right now. However, first thing in the morning, I must take Terror far away from here. I shall try to find a good owner or place for him. Terror is Lord Riley's best fighting dog. Lord Riley is not about to let Terror get away without making a huge effort to track him down so he can breed him some more and get him back into the pit."

Sir Thomas hugged Terror, "We can not allow that to happen, lest Terror be forced to fight to the death!" Sir Thomas looked in his uncle's eyes with great concern. "Is there anything I can do to help?"

Robert sighed before answering. "There is, though I do fear great danger for thee."

"Pray, tell me what must I do," Sir Thomas answered, unconcerned about himself.

"Take Terror somewhere at once!" Robert answered, uncertain that he was making the right decision involving his nephew. "Hide him just for tonight, without telling me where. Lord Riley will probably arrive here at any moment with the authorities to interrogate me on Terror's whereabouts. If I know, I may be forced to tell, for I cannot lie. If thou dost agree to this, we shall meet first thing in the morning, in back of church, right after the cock crows. From there, I shall take Terror from thee," Robert paused as a dark cold chill suddenly came upon him, "unless I am followed or some other form of complication should arise. In either case, I shall find thee."

Confused, Sir Thomas asked, "Uncle, how then would you find me?"

Robert looked over to Sly Ann. She looked back, wagging her tail. "Does that answer your question, nephew?"

"Indeed!" Sir Thomas responded, sighing and giving himself a quick slap to his forehead. "I should have known."

Robert, frightened for his nephew's wellbeing, patted Dare on the head, and said, "Pray, do promise me, nephew, that thou shalt listen to your dog by following his instincts, for he is thy guardian angel, and his instincts may keep thee alive!"

"With all due respect, I am Dare's master. He should obey me."

"Yes Nephew, I know thou art his master. Remember, though, what I did tell thee before. Dogs can sense what we cannot, so swear to me that thou shalt heed his instincts!"

*"So be it, I swear," Sir Thomas sighed as he did swear,*

*unaware of his uncle's scare, and on that note left with Terror and* Dare.

Sir Thomas did not take Terror to his own home for fear that Lord Riley might just show up there. Instead, he took Terror over to Charles' place. When Charles opened the door, he trembled with fear, for the first thing he saw was Terror sitting on his doorstep, staring at him. Sir Thomas calmed Charles down somewhat by explaining his situation and all that had happened. Pointing to Terror he said, "Go ahead Charles, thou canst pet him. He will not harm thee." Charles, still frightened, slowly extended his hand as Terror licked it. Charles began to pet Terror's head. Naturally, Charles agreed to help. He took Thomas and Terror to his stable and hid them there without telling his parents. That night after dinner, Charles snuck out to the barn with some food and blankets for them. It was a very good thing that Sir Thomas had left his uncle's house when he did, because immediately after he left, the authorities arrived, accompanied by Lord Riley, knocking on his uncle's door.

While Robert was opening his door, Lord Riley yelled, "Where the hell is my dog? Dognapper!"

Robert quickly answered in a calm tone of voice, "I am sorry, my Lord, but I do not know the whereabouts of your dog." Robert smiled because he was very pleased to see one of his former dogs accompanying his long time friend, Constable Jonathan Martin. The constable was also a very devout church member and regularly attended church on Sundays. Jonathan Martin had grown up with Robert and when they were both young, had mocked Robert's dogs. But after Jonathan grew up and became more mature and open-minded, he realized that Robert's dogs were by far the best working dogs around. That is why the constable was now the proud owner of one of Robert's dogs, and couldn't have been happier with any other dog.

After hearing Robert's statement, Constable Martin looked at Lord Riley, and told him confidently, "Your dog is not here." Then he turned to Robert with a big smile, and shook his hand, saying, "Hello mate."

Lord Riley was peeved at Constable Martin, and scolded him. "Sir, what do you mean, my dog is not here? This man is obviously lying. How dare you take his word for it?"

Constable Martin became angry in response. "Now you listen to me. First of all, I do not appreciate you raising your voice at me. Second, I have known Robert Gentry my whole life! There is no one I trust more than Robert and my mother. If Robert says that your dog is not here, then your dog is not here!" Knowing Constable Martin and Robert were friends, Lord Riley trembled with rage, but took several deep breaths to calm down.

While Lord Riley was restraining himself from exploding, Robert bent over to pet Constable Martin's dog. "How is Titus?"

Thumping Titus on his muscular chest, Jonathan replied, "He must be the strongest dog in the world, pound for pound! He doth make a fine Constable's dog. Several times he has helped me out in finding lost kids and bad people. I am most grateful that you gave him to me."

As Titus licked his face, Robert replied, "Tis my pleasure. I am glad to see him happy, and finding his calling in life."

Lord Riley changed his angry tone of voice to a calmer one as he spoke to Constable Martin. "Alright, so ye two are friends. That is splendid. However, I do have the right to get my dog back! So I plead, help search his premises for my dog."

Constable Martin looked at Lord Riley with an angry expression, and with both fists clenched by his waist. He was just about to scold Lord Riley again when Robert spoke up. "Tis alright, me mate; do let him search if it doth make him feel better. Ye are all more than welcome to search my entire property."

Constable Martin responded, "I am not searching. Thy word is good enough for me." Constable Martin pointed at Lord Riley, warning him, "If you damage any of Robert's possessions, I shall arrest you!"

Lord Riley responded, "As you say" with a quiet growl.

Lord Riley searched all around while Constable Martin and his partner sat down with Robert and had a nice conversation over some hot apple cider. When Lord Riley was finished looking for Terror, he walked back into Robert's house only to hear the two Constables laughing over one of Robert's dog stories. Robert began telling another story but was abruptly interrupted by Lord Riley. "I have searched the whole premises. Robert has my dog hidden somewhere else. I want him arrested now and put in jail until he tells where my dog is!"

Constable Martin chuckled as his partner replied, "We can not arrest a person based solely on accusations."

Lord Riley pointed at the cuts and bruises on his face, which he had received from Dare and from fighting with Robert. "Look you, then, at what this evil man did to my face! I cannot see anything out of my right eye! I do demand most strongly that he be arrested for assault!"

Constable Martin pointed at Lord Riley while telling him in an aggravated tone, "Now you listen to me! The fact that you are a filthy rich Lord does not make you my superior. I shall not heed your orders! I suggest that you shut your mouth and let Robert tell me what happened!" Constable Martin corrected himself, "Ah- I mean his side of the story!" Constable Martin looked at Robert. "Do proceed. We are listening. What happened? Didst thou attack Lord Riley?"

"I did hit Lord Riley, yes, I say. However, it was strictly in self defense; for you see, he did attack me first." (Robert pointed at his face where he was kicked.) "These are the bruises I received due to Lord Riley." Constable Martin and his partner didn't need to hear any more. Both of them looked at Lord Riley with narrowed eyes, an expression that insinuated, "You are a liar!"

Constable Martin warned Lord Riley, "Robert has an excellent reputation in town for being one of the most honest, kindest, caring, and giving persons. You, on the other hand, have the reputation of being a selfish, greedy, cruel, heartless dog fighter! However, if you want to waste a lot of people's time and look like an idiot by fighting Robert in court, you can. Keep in mind though, that God is on Robert's side. You may be the one spending time in jail yourself." Hearing this, Lord Riley turned red in the face with rage. He knew that the best thing he could do at this point was to get out of there fast, so he turned for the door and ran towards it. He couldn't see too well out of his right eye and tripped over a chair, landing flat on his face, and bruising it even more. After this happened, Constable Martin, his partner, and Robert laughed as Lord Riley quickly rose to his feet running out the door. Once outside, Lord Riley ran away from Robert's house as fast as he could. When he got a long distance away, Lord Riley yelled curses at the top of his lungs.

# CHAPTER XXXI
# LEGEND ON THE RUN

After Lord Riley released some of his frustrations, he went over to the manor of his cousin, Sherman III. Angrily, he knocked hard on the door. Vivian answered. "Good even, uncle-uh- did you get Terror back?"

Lord Riley knew that Vivian knew the answer and avoided the question. He was perturbed, and said, "I need to speak to my cousin."

At that moment, Sherman III walked into the room knowing exactly why his cousin had come over. He looked at his clock saying, "Son, 'tis getting late. 'Tis time for thee to go to bed." Sherman III did not want his son to hear him talking with his cousin about killing someone. Vivian didn't know that his father was an assassin. Nor did he want to go to bed. He was also upset about Terror running away. Vivian knew that his father and uncle were going to talk about trying to get Terror back and was curious how. So he asked, "Father, may I stay up? I am not sleepy."

Vivian's father didn't like repeating himself. He slapped his son across the face. "Does that answer your question?" After that, Vivian immediately went to his bedroom and did not say another word. Meanwhile, Sherman III walked over to his wall and took down his favorite sword while saying, "Young lads, like women, often need to be put in their place." Then while sticking his sword into a stuffed dummy used for practicing he went on to say, "I know why you came over here."

Lord Riley looked at his cousin with raging eyes. "The best fighting dog in history has been stolen from me, and is being corrupted and turned into a wimp as we speak."

Sherman III continued to strike the dummy, causing feather stuffing to fill the room. "I must say, 'twas rather shocking to see Terror let go of Dare and run off with Thomas and Dare. I did think that you trained Terror to be a mean killer, not one in which shows mercy to his foes."

Hearing this, Lord Riley clenched his fists in rage. "I did train Terror to be a killer! I do not know what happened! I do know though, that I must get him back before his appointed fight with Brahma the Bull! Otherwise, I do fear that I shall lose more money in one day than most people earn in a whole lifetime."

Sherman III took down another sword from the wall. "Fear not. I do promise that tomorrow thou shalt have thy dog back!"

Lord Riley watched with a closed smile as his cousin, using both swords at the same time, dramatically and skillfully sliced the dummy up into little pieces. "Robert claims that he does not know Terror's whereabouts, but he is lying, I know that he does know! I want that bastard to die a painful death unless he tells me where my favorite beast is!"

Sherman III put down his swords, and looked at his cousin confidently as he said, "I do promise! If your foe doth know where Terror is or who has him, he will tell! For no one is faithful enough to keep a secret to the point of suffering from one of my painful deaths," Sherman III paused with a chuckle, "Especially over something as unimportant as someone else's dog."

Lord Riley paced back and forth. "I am uncertain cousin, that Robert is crazy! He treats dogs as if they were humans."

"'Tis late now," Sherman III replied, yawning. "Let us get some sleep. Tomorrow morning, take me to where Robert lives and I shall make him talk."

That night, deep in thought, Robert sat by the fire with all his dogs gathered around. Lord Riley's enraged face remained in his brain. Robert knew Lord Riley was very disturbed about losing Terror. Big trouble was inevitable. Sly Ann saw Robert's troubled eyes staring at the fire. She also became troubled. She leaped in her master's lap, licking him in the face. Robert put two hands on Sly Ann's face, staring with a serious intense look deep into her eyes while saying, "Should anything happen to me tonight, I want thee to run to Dare, as fast as thou can. Warn him that great danger is coming their way and tell him to take care of my nephew at any cost and lead Terror far away to a safe place." Sly Ann couldn't understand Robert's words, but she understood his eyes. She rested her head on her master's shoulder as he held her in his arms while continuing to stare at the fire. Robert petted Sly Ann's head while praying, "Dear God, I pray for Lord Riley and everyone who abuses Thy most loving creatures. I ask Thee to soften their hearts; may they love innocent dogs half as much as Thee. Have mercy, I pray, on the dogs and on their abusers who hurt your precious creatures for sick entertainment. I pray that the abusers will feel a touch of the dog's pain that they inflict. Please watch over and protect my favorite nephew and my children, these dogs." Robert paused kissing Sly Ann on top of her head before finishing his prayer. "Also I do pray for my own protection, that I may be able to continue taking care of them, giving them back the love that they give." After praying thus, Robert fell asleep with Sly Ann in his arms as the fire slowly burned out.

The next morning before the sun rose and the rooster crowed, Lord Riley and Sherman III awoke. Before leaving, Lord Riley left a note for Vivian, telling him to tend his dogs and clean up their leavings, if he and Sherman

III weren't back soon. Sherman III brought his dog Fletcher, just in case Robert really didn't know where Terror was. Fletcher was short with heavy wrinkles and a long snout. He was the best tracking dog around. Fletcher could find anyone or anything days away as long as he had some fresh scent to go by. On their way to Robert's house, Lord Riley stopped by his place to get ten of his best fighting dogs, out of fear that Terror and Dare might be over at Robert's. Lord Riley knew the fighting ability of Terror and Dare, and he did not want to come into a confrontation with them without some serious backup. When they approached Robert's house early that morning, Sly Ann heard them. She woke up from a deep sleep, and jumped out of her masters lap barking. The rest of Robert's dogs woke up doing likewise. From a dead sleep, Robert leaped out of his chair to look out of his window and saw Lord Riley and Sherman III approaching, holding torches in their hands. Alongside of them were ten big, powerful, fighting dogs. Robert knew that he and his fast herding dogs were no match against them. He also knew that his dogs wouldn't think twice about sacrificing their lives for him, so he went outside, keeping his dogs inside and closing the door behind him, making sure that none of his dogs could get out. Robert knew that Lord Riley wanted Terror back at any cost, even if it meant Robert's life. Once outside Robert, ran his fastest trying to get to Bolt, his fastest horse. Robert was going to try to ride to safety and report Lord Riley to the authorities. Lord Riley saw Robert running, and while pointing at him, commanded his fastest dog Bruiser to attack. Robert made it all the way to Bolt. Robert jumped and was merely a fraction of a second away from sitting on Bolt and riding off to safety. Unfortunately, Bruiser also jumped at the same moment, and intercepted him. He bit Robert on the right shoulder while knocking him to the ground. Bruiser held Robert there, as Robert screamed in pain. Robert's dogs barked louder than they had ever done in their entire lives, trying desperately to get out of the house so they could come to their beloved master's defense, but they couldn't get out.

Lord Riley approached Robert with a sinister smile. "Well, look you what we have here. You would have been a lot better off had your stupid Constable mate arrested you and locked you in jail. However, I am willing to let bygones be bygones if you just give my dog back"

Robert, getting bitten by Bruiser on the leg, screamed out in pain, "Call your dog off!"

Lord Riley crossed his arms, unconcerned. "Not until you tell me where Terror is," Lord Riley said as he looked cautiously around and thought, *"At any moment, Terror and Dare shall appear with the rest of Robert's dogs in what shall surely be a bloody fight to the death."* Lord Riley wanted to make bloody sure that he got far away from that dogfight and found someplace to hide until it was over. Minutes passed, and Lord Riley was pleasantly surprised that none of Robert's dogs came to his defense. "'Tis much easier than I anticipated," Lord Riley commented, continuing to look around. "Where are your dogs? I do hear them barking, yet not one of them is coming to your defense. I did think that your dogs were much more devoted to you." Lord Riley commanded Bruiser, "Release him," then asked, "Are you ready to return Terror to me?"

Robert put his left hand on his knee, looking at the blood from Bruiser's bite. With tears in his eyes, he answered. "I do swear, I do not know Terror's whereabouts!"

Lord Riley and his cousin, each with arms crossed, shook their heads as they looked at Robert with uncompassionate eyes. "Wrong answer," Lord Riley replied. "Ares, Bruiser, attack!" Both huge dogs lunged at Robert, locking their jaws onto Robert's arms and crushing them.

Robert continued screaming out in pain. "Pray, make them stop! I swear I do not know!"

Sherman III looked down at Robert and spat on him. "'Tis most unfortunate!"

Lord Riley called more of his dogs. "Zeus, Hera, attack!" The two dogs attacked ripping, crushing Robert's skin and bones. "Are you now ready to talk?" Robert didn't answer. He continued screaming in pain as he fought the dogs. Lord Riley watched, shaking his head, "It does not have to be this way. Argo, Kara, attack." Lord Riley and Sherman III watched, every now and than exchanging baffled glances, each thinking, "How could anyone withstand so much pain? And to think it's over a dumb dog!" As the dogs attacked, Robert's bones could be heard breaking. Lord Riley called his dogs off. "I shall now ask you one more time! Where is Terror?"

Robert knew at this point that he had no chance of survival. The sooner he died, the better off he would be. He whispered, "Come here."

Lord Riley bent over, "Yes, go ahead, tell me!"

Robert whispered again, "Come closer," Lord Riley bent over even closer. Robert whispered really quietly, "Terror is at . . . "

Lord Riley enthusiastically replied, "Tell me," with his ear a half an inch away from Robert's mouth. Lord Riley thought for sure that he was about to be told Terror's whereabouts. But much to his surprise, Robert lunged forward with his head, biting him on the ear. Robert violently shook his head back and forth, as Lord Riley bled, screaming out in pain. "Get him the bloody hell off of me!" Sherman III quickly pulled out his razor sharp sword.

As Robert bit off a small piece of Lord Riley's ear, spitting it far away, Sherman III sliced through his neck with his sword, separating head from body. Lord Riley put his hand over his bloody ear, screaming out, "That bloody bastard bit my ear!" His cousin held a torch up to Lord Riley's ear and noticed that a piece had been bitten off. He cut off a piece of Robert's shirt that didn't have any blood on it, took out his wine, and poured it on his cousin's ear to prevent infection. Then he had his cousin hold the piece of Robert's shirt up to his ear to help stop the bleeding. While they were doing this, Bruiser attacked Robert's headless body, ripping and tearing away at the flesh.

The two men, along with Fletcher, looked around for the small piece of ear. Sherman III soon gave up. "Let us stop now, cousin. 'Tis like looking for a needle in a haystack. 'Twill soon be light. I do fear Robert's Constable friend will soon come by to check on him." Sherman III paused sighing, thinking about the consequences if he were caught with Robert's fresh blood on him: a noose around his throat. Sherman III finished by saying, "We must not be caught with bloody hands by Robert's Constable friend."

Lord Riley didn't stop, but desperately continued to search with Fletcher. "What if someone finds a piece of my ear here? I shall surely be charged with murder and hanged to death."

"With all thy money," Sherman III replied with a slight chuckle, "thou couldst probably buy thy way free. Besides, if Fletcher cannot find thine ear, no one else shall be able to do so, either!" Hearing this, Lord Riley calmed down a little and sat down on a log.

Sherman III put his torch down, and took out a needle and some thread, which he had brought just in case there might be an injury that required stitches. Next Sherman III had his cousin hold the torch up high near his face, as he began stitching up the ear.

Out of the corner of his eye, Lord Riley watched Bruiser, who was still tearing away at Robert's flesh. "Such a pitiful shame he bit my ear," Lord Riley said, addressing Bruiser. "Otherwise I would have had the extreme pleasure of watching thee eat his bloody flesh while he was still alive!"

Sherman III shook his head, saying about Bruiser, "That is one possessed beast thou hast."

"My thanks for the compliment. Bruiser's merciless nature is the standard for how all my dogs should be."

Sherman III smiled as he continued to stitch. He chuckled, "Thou art one demented bastard."

Robert's dogs continued biting away at the shutters, trying desperately to get out so they could run to their master's defense. They were almost free as Sherman III finished stitching. "That should stop your bleeding," he said proudly, helping Lord Riley up with his hand. Without remorse, the two looked at Robert's head on the ground. "Let us now get out of here, go over to Sir Thomas', find that bloody bastard and do likewise to him!" Sherman III paused giving an arrogant smirk. "Soon thou shalt have thy dog back." They picked up their things and left.

A few seconds after they had left, Robert's dogs bit through the closed and locked shutters, then jumped out and ran over to their headless master. Gathering around, they cried out in agony. With his teeth, Blaze picked up his master's head by the hair, carried it back over to his master's mangled body, then tried desperately to put it back together again. Robert's blood cried out to Sly Ann, reminding her of what he wanted her to do. Quickly, she held her howls, and pulled herself together. She turned her head, seeing the shirt that Sir Thomas had giving her master the day before. She walked over to it. The shirt still had Sir Thomas's scent on it. Sly Ann took a big whiff, then took off running faster than she ever had in her entire life, towards Sir Thomas. She knew Terror and Dare would also be there.

Sly Ann ran, howling out, "Great danger is approaching your way!" Dare soon awoke to Sly Ann's desperate howls, understanding exactly what his little friend was warning about. He cuffed his jaws with his lips as he wrapped his mouth around Thomas' head. Gently he pulled so his master safely awoke in a sitting position.

Once awake, Sir Thomas asked, "What is the matter, thou mad beast?" Dare barked, pacing back and forth. Sir Thomas knew that something was definitely wrong and understood that his dog wanted to leave immediately. Sir Thomas put on his shoes, rose to his feet, and left Charles' barn with Terror and Dare. As they left, Sir Thomas could faintly hear Sly Ann in the distance. He looked at Terror and Dare as he said, "That doth sounds like Sly Ann. Something might be the matter with my uncle. We need to go check on him." Sir Thomas tried walking towards his uncle's home, but as he did, both dogs barked ferociously, blocking his way and preventing him from heading there. Sir Thomas remembered swearing to his uncle about obeying Dare, so reluctantly he complied, saying, "Alright, I will follow ye two mad beasts! Lead the way." Terror and Dare knew that Lord Riley had killed Sir Thomas' uncle and would stop at nothing to getting Terror back. They also knew that Lord Riley had a lot of help.

Dare raised his head in the air, giving a loud howl which meant, "Thanks for the warning, Sly Ann. I understand and am very sorry about your master. Return home now. My master will be taken care of, and I am prepared to kill for him. I shall guard him with my life and with every fiber of my being." Hearing Dare's reply, Sly Ann knew her master's request had been granted. She turned around and returned home, where she sat next to her master with her head pointing up high. Sly Ann loved her master with all of her heart. In terrible agony, she howled aloud over his death as Terror and Dare led Sir Thomas in the direction of Hell Hound Forest.

# CHAPTER XXXII
# BROKEN PROMISE

The fog was very thick that morning. Sir Thomas, seeing Terror and Dare heading towards a place that was strictly forbidden, spoke up. "We cannot continue in this direction!"

Dare responded by walking in back of his master, barking as if to say, "Yes we are, and you are coming with us!" Sir Thomas ignored the barks and walked passed them. "Terror and I are going to meet my uncle in back of church, as planned. Come Terror!" Dare barked even louder, reminding his master of his promise.

Sir Thomas turned around and said, "Yes Dare, I know I swore to my uncle that I would listen to thee. But I also swore a long time ago never to go near Hell Hound Forest. Besides, my uncle may be in danger and may need our help!" Terror ran in front of Sir Thomas, growling and exposing his massive fangs. Sir Thomas knew for a fact that Dare would never harm him, but he wasn't certain that Terror, who was also now starting to growl, wouldn't bite him. Besides, Sir Thomas had promised his uncle that he would listen to Dare. "Alright," Sir Thomas said, frustrated, and changed his direction. "Ye two win. I shall follow the two of ye. As long as ye do not become possessed with a Hell Hound spirit, which as was written long ago, is what happens to dogs who come here." Dare responded by looking at his master, eyes crazed and with a snarl. "'Tis not funny," Sir Thomas said, not amused, as they began their journey into Hellhound Forest.

Meanwhile, Lord Riley with his retinue arrived at Sir Thomas' house. Sherman III knocked on the door while Lord Riley and the dogs stayed hidden. Sir Thomas' father answered the door, yawning and rubbing his eyes from being awakened. "Yes, may I help you?"

"Good day," Sherman III replied, extending his hand and shaking hands with Sir Thomas' father. He gave an alias, saying, "Stuart Ulrich is my name. I presume you are the father of one Sir Thomas Gentry?"

"Yes, that is correct."

"I must say, your son spoke rather highly of you. I do hope I did not awaken you."

"Tis alright. I had to get up in any event to answer the door," Mr. Gentry responded, pulling back his long, tangled hair. "How may I help you?"

"I came here to pay your son four shillings for cleaning up my yard."

With a suspicious look in his eyes, Sir Thomas' father answered, "'Tis rather odd. My son has been very busy lately. I had no idea he was doing side work for anyone."

"Oh dear! Sherman III said putting his hand over his mouth. "I may have really made a mess of things this time. He worked for me to earn money to buy a present for someone. I hope it was not you."

Sir Thomas' father smiled because his birthday happened to be in a couple of weeks. He thought, *"My wonderful son is working hard to earn money to buy me a nice birthday gift. I am proud of him!"* He responded, "My son is not here right now. He spent the night at his uncle's. You might want to try again later, or I can give him the four shillings."

"My thanks for the offer, Mr. Gentry. However, I do wish to see your son's face when he receives an extra ten pence for his superb work," Sherman III said, backing up with a confused expression as he thought, *"If Thomas spent the night at his uncle's, I wonder why he did not come out with his dogs to help defend his uncle?"*

Sir Thomas' father yawned again. "I shall let my son know you were here."

"Thank you," replied Sherman III as he raised his hand and waved goodbye. He started to head back to his cousin when a pair of Sir Thomas' shoes near the front porch caught the corner of his eye. "Wait a moment," he mumbled, stopping abruptly. Once Mr. Gentry closed his door, Sherman III walked over and picked up one of the shoes. He placed the shoe in front of Fletcher's nose and said enthusiastically, "Go get it!" Fletcher took a big sniff of Sir Thomas' shoe, then lifted his head up high and looked side to side. His tail and ears rose up as he locked on to the scent of Sir Thomas. Fletcher then started heading in the direction where Sir Thomas was, with Sherman III following closely behind. Smiling confidently, he told his cousin, "As I said before, thou shalt get thy dog back!" They soon ended up at Hell Hound Forest. Faint howls were heard in the distance.

"I have no intentions of going on any farther." Lord Riley said, stopping. He felt an eerie chill run through his spine. "There have been several stories of Hell Hounds guarding this forest and devouring all who enter!"

Sherman III laughed. "Thou must be joking! Those are superstitious myths which were told a long time ago by some of the town crackpots. Hounds of Hell or Dogs of Doom do not exist! The dogs we heard are probably Terror and Dare trying to scare us!" At that moment, Fletcher froze, standing completely still. He lifted his head up, locking onto a disturbing scent that was influencing him to bark with fear. Fletcher turned completely around and ran in the opposite direction, wanting to get far away from Hell Hound Forest. Sherman III stopped Fletcher by slapping his head. "Onward, cowardly dog!"

he commanded. "Thou hast ten fighting dogs and us to protect you." The ten dogs didn't bark or turn around. However, their tails all stood straight up, signaling that they were troubled by something in the forest.

As they continued on, Lord Riley walked in the midst of his ten fighting dogs. Although he couldn't see any thing unusual, he could feel the presence of unwelcoming eyes upon him. Lord Riley constantly moved his head side to side, as he looked around, fearing that at any second a ghost dog might come flying at him from out of the fog. Sensing his cousin's fear, Sherman III, mocked him. "I do say, perhaps we should turn around, for nobody has shed more innocent dog's blood than thee! If there is any truth to the myth, we both are surely doomed."

*Sherman the Third's words had described Lord Riley's thoughts to a tee,*
*yes it was true nobody had shed more dog's blood than he.*
*Lord Riley quivered and shivered as he stared at the moon,*
*sensing his fate may be soon.*

Sir Thomas also heard faint howls in the distance. "That is it," he said convinced. "We are turning around and going home! My father would not spare the rod if he knew I was out here. I now command both of ye to come home with me!" Terror and Dare didn't budge. "So be it," Sir Thomas said annoyed. "I shall go home alone!" Terror and Dare watched Sir Thomas take twenty steps towards home, before fearfully freezing dead in his tracts. At that moment, the forest was filled with loud howls and odd noises. Sir Thomas quickly turned around, running back to Terror and Dare. He had now gone too far. There was no way he was going to leave the two best fighting dogs on the planet and walk half way through Hellhound forest alone. "Alright!" Sir Thomas said running to catch up. "Ye two jesters win! I shall go with ye." The two brothers both knew that Sir Thomas wasn't going to go far without them. Continuing on, Sir Thomas stayed in the middle, his hands on both dog's backs, his head moving from side to side as he cautiously looked around. Meanwhile, that morning Constable Jonathan Martin had decided to stop by his friend Robert's place to check and make sure that Lord Riley didn't cause any more problems. When Jonathan came within a half mile of Robert's place, he heard all of Robert's dogs howling in great distress. Hearing this, Jonathan rode his horse faster. When he arrived, he found his friend Robert dead in a pool of blood, with all of his dogs gathered around.

As he jumped off his horse, Jonathan cursed Lord Riley's name. He cried alongside Robert's dogs, shouting out, "Why? How couldst thou allow this, Lord?" After this outburst Jonathan dried his tears, mumbling with Lord Riley's face planted in his brain.

"You shall pay, Lord Riley! I do not yet know how, but you shall."

Sly Ann stopped howling for the moment. She lifted her nose up in the air, smelling an unusual scent coming from the spot where she had taken a piss in the night, shortly before Lord Riley and Sherman III showed up. She walked over to the spot and found the missing piece of Lord Riley's ear, which her master had spit out after he had bitten it off. The reason Fletcher hadn't been able to smell the ear was that it had landed in the little puddle created by Sly Ann's urine, which had hidden the scent of the ear. Now the urine had dried, making it easier for Sly Ann to smell the ear. She picked up the piece of ear in her mouth and brought it over to Jonathan, who carefully took it out of her mouth. His eyes opened up with great surprise as he patted Sly Ann on the head. "Good girl Sly Ann! Good girl! We are going to get that bloody bastard now! I would wager anything that this piece of ear belongs to Lord Riley. I shall take great pleasure in watching him hang. I shall also bring thee and all of Robert's dogs to see the hanging." Jonathan carefully wrapped the ear up and rode his fastest toward his superiors, to report the news. Afterwards, he and his partner Carl went to Sir Thomas' home to tell his parents the bad news. Immediately, they cried, holding one another.

"Where is my son?" Mrs. Gentry screamed out, terrified. She paused looking at her husband, "He spent last night at your brother's!"

Hearing this, Jonathan and Carl exchanged worried looks as Jonathan answered, "We do not know of his whereabouts. Nobody was found there except for Robert."

Hearing this, Mrs. Gentry screamed out panic-stricken. "I want my son! Find him!"

Carl responded in a calm and reassuring tone of voice, "We will do our very best to find your son. Is there any information either of you can give that may help?"

"NO!" Mrs. Gentry cried out.

While crying, Mr. Gentry nodded his head yes, closing his eyes tightly to control his tears as he answered. "A strange man came by early this morning, whom I had never seen before." Jonathan and Carl exchanged surprised glances.

"Oh, that does sounds rather odd. Can you describe this strange man?" asked Carl.

Mr. Gentry placed his hand on his chin, thinking a moment. "He is about forty years old, has dark brown hair, thick eyebrows, and distinct sideburns in a form of swords. He is slender and about six feet tall. He said his name was Stuart Ulrich."

Jonathan and Carl looked at each other, both saying at the same time, " Sherman III!" Jonathan turned to Mr. Gentry. "The person you described fits the description of a man named Sherman III. He probably gave you a false name. However, we shall comb our records for information about Stuart Ulrich."

Upset, Mr. Gentry responded, "I presume Sherman III is related to Lord Riley?"

Constable Martin nodded his head. "Indeed. Sherman III is Lord Riley's younger cousin and is even more evil. He has been suspected of murdering people in the past. Unfortunately, there has never been any proof." Hearing this, Mrs. Gentry cried out even louder as Jonathan asked, "Was that person bleeding at all from his ear, or did he have a cut on it?"

"No," Mr. Gentry answered."

"Is there anything else you can tell us?" asked Carl. Mr. Gentry shook his head no.

Jonathan looked around the yard. "Do you have anything with your son's scent, so we can give it to our hounds to help find your son?" Spotting Sir Thomas' shoe, Jonathan suggested, "Perhaps this shoe over here."

Mr. Gentry nodded yes, as he cried, holding his wife again.

Mrs. Gentry looked petrified at Jonathan as he walked over to pick up her son's shoe. "Where is the other shoe? 'Twas right next to that one!" Mrs. Gentry cried out. After hearing this, Jonathan and his partner didn't waste any more time. They knew that Lord Riley and Sherman III had the other shoe and were tracking down Sir Thomas in an attempt to get Terror back. Jonathan and Carl leaped on their horses, waving goodbye as they headed back for more help to find Sir Thomas.

As they rode off Mrs. Gentry screamed, "FIND MY SON!"

A minute later, Charles, Emily, Sara and their two dogs walked up and were greatly concerned to see Thomas' parents in tears. Seeing the young people, Mr. Gentry quickly blurted out, "Have you seen our son? He spent last night at my brother's place."

Emily and Sara exchanged confused glances, each thinking, *"So, what is the fuss about?"*

Mr. Gentry, seeing the exchanged glances and knowing their thoughts, looked away from them and towards the ground. His eyes gushed tears as he said, "I regret terribly to say that my brother was found murdered this morning." (Emily and Sara instantly cried like babies at hearing this.) "My wife and I fear the worst could be for our son."

Charles held his head to one side as tears gushed. Slowly he lifted his head up, responding. "I am confident that nothing bad has happened to your son. Last night, your brother told Sir Thomas to hide somewhere with Terror and Dare. Robert feared that trouble was inevitable at his place. Therefore, your son came over to my home last night. I snuck him and the two dogs into the barn."

Hearing this, Mrs. Gentry grabbed Charles by the shoulders. "Where is my son now?"

"Unfortunately, I do not know. This morning, when I opened the door of the stable where they slept last night, they were gone." On a good note Charles added, "I do know for a fact, though, that they left of their own free will."

Mr. Gentry dried his eyes with his hands, commenting while looking at the hills. "Somewhere out there, my son is alive and well, I can feel it. If Lord Riley is lucky, he will be arrested before Dare gets hold of him, lest the wrath of our family be bestowed upon him through Dare.

# CHAPTER XXXIII
# MEDIEVAL TORTURE

Sir Thomas, Terror, and Dare hiked all day through hellhound forest. They were extremely hungry. Thomas commented, "If I do not get something to eat soon, I am afraid I will die!" Just before the sun went down, Terror and Dare smelt the droppings of wild boar. They followed the scent until they found a family of ten. Quietly, Terror and Dare crept up behind the boar on each side, creating a surprise attack. They ganged up on the biggest one. Together they quickly killed the boar. They shared the boar, eating close together just like when they were little puppies. Very hungry, Sir Thomas reached towards the kill. "My thanks, I will take a little pi-," before Sir Thomas could say piece and grab any of the wild boar. Terror and Dare both growled at him, knowing Sir Thomas would become awfully ill if he ate any of the raw boar, unlike them. Sir Thomas hearing the growls and seeing both dogs' huge fangs pulled his hand quickly away. "Fine, thou savage beasts! Do not share any of thy boar with me. I shall just starve to death." Deep down inside though, he knew the dogs were keeping him away from the boar for his best interest.

Sir Thomas had learned from his father how to make a fire. As the two dogs ate, Sir Thomas gathered some sticks and wood together and soon made himself a nice little fire. After Sir Thomas did this, Dare ripped off a nice big chunk of flesh from the Boar and carried it over to his master with his mouth, "My thanks mate," Sir Thomas said as his dog put the piece of boar near him on a rock. Sir Thomas found a nice stick, put the flesh of boar on it and cooked it medium well, then indulged. Afterwards all three were full. They all snuggled up next to the fire together.

Fletcher came across the Boar droppings about a half an hour after Terror and Dare did.

Sherman III, seeing the droppings, knew that the boar were not far away. Rubbing his stomach he said, "I am hungry! Fletcher, find boar." It didn't take Fletcher long before he found the family of boar. Sherman III and Lord Riley watched the boar through some thick bushes. Lord Riley wanted to wait until the boar came a little closer to them before he sent his dogs for the kill. Bruiser however, ignorantly took off after the boar a little too early, followed by the rest of Lord Riley's dogs. The boars were all frightened and scattered away. Because of the dogs' failure, Sherman III became disgusted and angry because they had almost had what looked like a nice, easy meal.

Holding Sir Thomas' shoe, which he had stolen earlier, up to Fletcher 's nose he said again, "Go find" as he glared at his cousin, taking out his hunger charged frustrations. "I know why you want Terror back so badly; the rest of your so called bulldogs are worthless! Terror would have done better all by himself!"

Irritated, Lord Riley interrupted his cousin by grabbing his right shoulder. "Do not call my bulldogs worthless, for they have done very well for me in the pit, making me a rich lord!"

Sherman III swatted his cousin's hand away, "Get thy sorry bulldog hand off of me! Thy dogs may have made thee a lot of money. Terror, however, made thee more money in one fight than all thy sorry so-called bulldogs combined. If thou wouldst get Terror back and avoid a bloody beating, I do most strongly suggest that thou dost shut the bloody hell up." Lord Riley didn't say another word. He knew that his cousin was hungry and would make good on his threat. They continued searching for boar for another twenty more minutes before darkness settled over Hell Hound Forest.

It was extremely cold that night. Sir Thomas stood shivering close to the fire that he had made. Knowing that his master needed to be warmed and sleeping, Dare tugged with his teeth on his master's shirt, pulling it part way off. "What art thou doing? Thou art a mad beast!" Sir Thomas said unaware of his dog's plan. "Dost thou wish me to freeze to death?" Dare continued tugging on his master's shirt until Sir Thomas realized that his dog wanted to warm him up with body heat. "Alright," Sir Thomas said taking off his shirt. "I do believe I know what thou dost wish to do." Dare took his master's shirt and with his mouth, placed it flat on the ground in back of his master. Gently he pushed his master to the ground with his paw. Next, Dare and Terror snuggled on opposite sides of Sir Thomas, covering him up and making a body blanket for him. Both dogs gently rested their heads on the sides of Sir Thomas' face, leaving a passage for him to breathe through.

Meanwhile, about a mile away Lord Riley and Sherman III were trying to get settled for the night. Sherman III unwrapped the blanket that he had brought. The two lay down as Sherman III covered them.

"'Tis freezing out here!" Lord Riley said shivering. "I would not be the least bit surprised if we found Sir Thomas frozen to death tomorrow. He is probably hungrier and colder than both of us combined!"

Feeling his hunger pangs, Sherman III replied, "Do not remind me about being hungry. I am still angry with thee and thy so-called bulldogs for not catching us food." At that very moment, Sir Thomas was snoring away with his two big buddies snuggled up close keeping him nice and warm. All three were full.

*Lord Riley and Sherman III on the other hand, resentfully snuggled close shaking like leaves on a tree, hungry as can be, not sleeping easily.*

That night, Sir Thomas' parents snuggled up next to the fire, holding each other, hoping and praying for the safe return of their son and Dare.

Mrs. Gentry cried and cried, "Where is my son? I want him back."

Mr. Gentry put his hand on her face. "Try not to worry my dear; our son is alright. He is in the best hands and paws possible. Besides being under Dare's care, our son is also in God's hands, and if God be for us, who can be against us?"

Hearing this, Mrs. Gentry calmed down a little, replying. "I do hope so."

Mr. Gentry closed his eyes and kissed her head. "He is." Mr. Gentry went on to say. "My brother Robert is now an angel watching over us right now as we speak."

Mrs. Gentry began to cry many tears again, saying. "I love our son more than life itself. He is so young. I hate to imagine what life would be without him."

Mr. Gentry put his chest next to his wife's head, enfolding his wife's head in his arms. "I know this is not easy, but everybody has suffered catastrophes in their lives at one time or another. This happens to be our toughest yet by far. We must embrace this pain, keep our faith and be strong." Mr. Gentry said this as he cried like a baby himself. He even began losing faith and fearing the worst for their son.

Early the next morning, before the sun rose, Sherman III woke his cousin and the dogs. "Come on, time to get up." He said emphatically, "Sir Thomas and Terror are not far away from us. If we leave now, we might be able to get them before they awake, and so catch Terror in my net."

Lord Riley forced himself to his feet from a terrible night's sleep. His nose ran from a cold that he had begun to come down with. "'Twould be great if we could catch Terror before he awakens. That way I could bring him back uninjured and in good shape for his fight against Brahma the Bull in a few weeks."

Sherman III responded, chuckling, "Not to mention, thy ten best fighting dogs would probably not be able to defeat Terror and Dare, without help from my swords!"

Lord Riley swallowed, thinking about this for a second before replying. "Together, these ten dogs will be able to defeat Terror and Dare, without help from thy swords!"

"Ha, dost thou want to put thy money where thy mouth is?"

Deep down inside, Lord Riley wasn't sure. He weaseled out of the bet. "I shall never bet against my best fighting dog."

"Yes, thou wouldst, were there money for thee to make." After hearing this accurate statement, Lord Riley kept his mouth shut.

Fletcher led them about a mile before they saw the dying embers of the fire Sir Thomas had made and the remainders of the boar Terror and Dare caught.

Seeing this, Sherman III slapped his cousin upside the head, mockingly whispering his cousin's own words. "I do wager that Sir Thomas is twice as hungry as we are," he said, slapping him again. "It does not look like it there, now does it? I do wager he is still full and probably," (at that moment Sherman III saw the two dogs snuggled up with Sir Thomas) "nice and warm and having a good night sleep, unlike us, who are both tired and starving," Sherman III raised his hand. He restrained himself from slapping again for fear of waking up Terror and Dare. He continued by whispering mockingly, "I would not be surprised if we found Sir Thomas frozen to death tomorrow! Thou art lucky thou art my cousin."

Sherman III and Lord Riley quietly opened up the net, creeping up along side Terror and Dare. Just when they were next to them, Dare heard them and woke up. He raised his head as Sherman III screamed, "NOW!" As the net was coming down, Dare shoved his master with all fours, causing him to fly seven feet in the air and land just outside the net. Terror and Dare sprang up, trying to escape the net. Unfortunately, both of them were about a quarter of a second to late. They each were tangled up on opposite sides of the net, near the ends. Dare looked at his master and barked as if to say, "Run master, run." However, Sir Thomas had no intentions of leaving these two dogs behind. Sherman III and Lord Riley laughed as they jumped, slapping one another's hands in celebration.

Lord Riley soon calmed down a little and wiped the buggers from his nose, caused by the cold that he had now come down with in earnest. He looked over at Sir Thomas, who was glancing over at Dare. "I know just what thou art thinking right now," Lord Riley said proud of his capture. "Thou art thinking about setting thy dog free so he could defend thee like he did against Bulldread." Lord Riley shook his head no, as he continued, "That will not happen this time. One false move and Bruiser will tear thee apart where thou dost stand." Bruiser growled as his name was mentioned. Lord Riley moved his eyes onto Terror, speaking with concern and with open palms. "Why hast thou forsaken me? Thou dost have no idea how frightened I was about losing thee, or by being forced to use ten of my best fighting dogs against thee!" In a suddenly harsh and unsympathetic tone, Lord Riley went on to say. "Thou hast no idea how much money is at stake for me over your next fight in a few weeks! I need thee healthy and strong so thou canst put on a good show before thou dost die in the pit." Lord Riley turned his eyes back to Sir Thomas. "I have whipped Terror! Beaten him! Made him watch other dogs eat dinner while he had none and had to go to sleep hungry! Treated him more mean and cruel than any animal ever has been treated. For a long time, he lived up to his name and was known as the meanest son of a bitch on the planet!" (Lord Riley turned his eyes to Dare, who continued barking to try to warn his master to leave.) "Thou shouldst have listened to your dog. He has good instincts. He knows that his master is about to die!" Lord Riley's scary evil eyes slowly shifted back over to Sir Thomas. "Before I kill thee, I want to know how thou didst change Terror into being merciful, sparing your life and Dare's."

Sir Thomas stared deep into Lord Riley's eyes, answering. "All the abuse you have done over the years can not compare to the powerful love that Dare and I have shown him."

Sherman III chuckled as he mocked Sir Thomas. "Love will not protect thee now

from being killed!" Seeing the power of love Sir Thomas had in his eyes, Lord

Riley looked away feeling uneasy. He walked over to Bruiser, and put his hand

on Bruiser's head, tapping with his fingers. "Thou dost certainly look hungry," Lord

Riley said, glaring at Sir Thomas. Lord Riley took hold of Bruiser, grabbing his skin

and crunching it up in his hand before shouting, "KILL!" Bruiser took off charging as

Lord Riley moved his arm along with Bruiser, helping him get a quicker jump. Seeing

Bruiser charging over to Sir Thomas in hungry, angry killing mode, Terror and Dare

desperately tried to get free, but to no avail.

Sherman III laughed, mocking again by saying, "Let us see the power of love save thee now." Just then, out of the fog, a fast, agile, and powerful female dog showed up, springing at Bruiser's throat and locking on. Bruiser came within one inch of biting Sir Thomas. The female dog ferociously shook her head back and forth. Bruiser's neck spurted blood everywhere, some of it even landing in the faces of Sherman III and Lord Riley, who stood watching with their mouths open in awe. Bruiser's head was eventually torn off. The female dog swung Bruiser's head in the air towards Lord Riley, and it hit him right in the testicles, causing a bloody mess, and making Lord Riley keel over. This dog looked even meaner than Terror did when he was corrupted.

The female dog stared deep into Lord Riley's eyes. Her face and teeth dripped with the blood from Bruiser's throat. Her massive, powerful jaws and razor sharp teeth were fully exposed, just waiting for Lord Riley to make a move.

*Lord Riley, now a firm believer in the Hounds of Hell,*
*froze like a dead man as he listened for the reaper's bell.*
*Carefully he looked at this dog who mysteriously came out of the fog.*
*Her powerful ripping muscles resembled Terror and Dare's,*
*even her massive jaws resembled theirs.*
*Lord Riley noticing distinct spots of brindle markings on her back,*
*mumbled, having a flashback.*

"I remember thee when thou wert just a little pup. Thou art no Hound of Hell, but merely Terror and Dare's sister."

Sherman III, hearing his cousin's mumbled words, looked over at Terror and Dare. He could clearly see the resemblance between them and this female dog. "Oh! Is that it?" Sherman III said while taking out his two favorite swords, one with each hand. "For a moment, I was even starting to believe in the ludicrous stories of the Hounds of Hell!" Just then Terror and Dare broke free and stood next to their long lost sister, foaming at the mouth, their jaws fully exposed. Seeing this, Lord Riley once again had a look of fear on his face.

Sherman III smiled and said, "Do calm down, cousin. We have nine fighting dogs plus Fletcher, as well as my two swords" (Sherman III impressively waved his swords around in the air) "with which I am very skilled. There is no way that these three dogs can defeat us." Just then a powerful and gigantic male dog appeared out of the fog from behind a tree and stood next to Terror and Dare's sister. This dog was her mate, the dog that saved her life after Lord Riley had abandoned to die in the forest. Seeing this new dog (which was bigger than any dog he had ever seen), Sherman III was troubled. "Well, we still out number them. Give thy dogs the command to attack."

Lord Riley didn't say a word, but fearfully looked in disbelief. Even his fighting dogs were scared of these four dogs. They growled, ready to fight, but knew that in fighting, their lives would come to an end. They saw how Bruiser's head had been severed from his body and knew that he was the best fighter of the ten. They also knew Terror's extraordinary fighting ability and inner strength.

Sherman III, ready to start swinging his swords at the dogs, nudged his cousin with his shoulder. "Proceed! Command thy dogs to attack!" Lord Riley opened his mouth and was about to give the command, but held his tongue, for he saw seven more dogs with heads hung low slither out from the fog. The seven dogs' fangs were fully exposed, welcoming a fight. The dogs walked over to Terror and Dare's sister; they were her offspring that had just turned two years old. Four females and three males all had developed into powerful creatures, which looked like freaks of nature. Seeing this, Lord Riley's eyes bulged even more than before. Slowly he backed away with his dogs and Sherman III.

Sir Thomas, seeing this, raised both hands in the air saying, "My thanks, God, for sending nine archangels to our rescue." Sir Thomas, noticing Sherman III backing up and contemplating using his swords, shook his head no as a warning while pointing his finger at him. "Ah, I would strongly advise against doing that!" Sherman III heeded the warning and slowly put his swords to his sides in surrender.

Lord Riley kept slowly backing up, mumbling, "Call them off and we will do whatever you ask of us." However, on the inside he was thinking, "When these dogs are away, I am going to personally slice thee into a thousand bloody little pieces!"

Sir Thomas paced back and forth, in back of Dare and his allies as he demanded, "Give your dogs their own free will, to leave you if they so please."

Lord Riley with his hands up in surrender nodded yes as he replied. "Alright, if they want to leave they may."

Sir Thomas enthusiastically responded with a huge smile while addressing Lord Riley's nine dogs.

*"Did you hear what your master just said?*
*He is giving permission to be free if you want to be.*
*No longer must you live in captivity.*
*Therefore I say, run away,*
*your whole life's been led astray!*
*Go I say, run away!*
*No longer must you kill against your will!*
*Run away I say,*
*be free, see what wonders lie in store for thee,*
*run away I say,*
*no longer must you mirror after your evil master.*
*Therefore I say, run away,*
*before you bear pain by Terror and Dare, and die in vain.*
*Go now, one more time I say, run away."*

After Sir Thomas spoke these words, the nine dogs slowly turned, glancing at one another, then over at Lord Riley one last time with sad eyes as they thought, *"We loved and served you for years, even after you continually abused us, never showing any compassion. How could any creature be so cold?"* The dogs turned their backs on Lord Riley and took off running, as he screamed, "No! Do not go! For I am nothing without you! Come back!" As Lord Riley yelled this, Dare's sister crouched back ready to spring at him. She was literally going to tear his heart out that moment and would have if not for Dare who barked requesting her not to just yet.

Sherman III was now horrified. He told his cousin, "Shut up and do not move! We both do know what these beasts are capable of doing!"

Sir Thomas smiled, waving goodbye at the nine dogs as they ran away free. When they were gone, he turned to Lord Riley and mocked him, saying, "Those dogs were nothing with you." Lord Riley's eyes filled with rage from hearing this smart-aleck remark and seeing his best fighting dogs run away. Dare along, with the rest of the dogs, saw the rage in Lord Riley's eyes. This influenced all of them to bark, growl and foam at the mouth even more. Lord Riley knew that they could tell what he was thinking from looking in his eyes. Therefore, he closed his eyes in an attempt to hide his rage. He mumbled with a big phony smile that showed with all his bright white teeth, "Sir Thomas, please tell these kind dogs to back off and leave us alone."

Sir Thomas responded with his hand to his chin, "Hmm, if I ask them to leave you alone, will you swear on both the Holy Bible and your mother's grave to leave Terror alone, letting him go wherever he so desires to roam?"

Lord Riley kept his eyes closed, and his teeth ground together with a phony smile as he answered. "Of course I will swear on the Holy Bible and my mother's grave, for I care very much about Terror's feelings. If he wants to leave me, so be it." The words, though, which were really in Lord Riley's heart when he said these lies were, *"You bloody little bastard! Terror is my slave. He makes me rich by fighting in the pit! Once your pathetic naive little arse falls for my phony vows, I shall kill thee with my own two hands! "*

"Will you also swear on the Holy Bible and your mother's grave never to bother my uncle or any of our dogs again? Before you make this vow, open your eyes and look in mine." The moment Lord Riley opened his eyes, the dogs crouched back, furiously barking.

Lord Riley's voice rumbled with fear, "Of course I promise. Now call these dogs off."

Sir Thomas rubbed his chin with his index finger, deep in thought. *"By the way all these dogs are barking and the look in Lord Riley's eyes, I question his honesty. However, what choice do I have? For Lord Riley is a rich, powerful Lord. If these dogs attack and kill him, the finest authorities will be put on his case. They shall surely track him down and find he and his cousin's bitten up corpses. The authorities will be able to prove by the teeth marks that Dare participated. In which he will instantly be killed and I may be charged with murder.*" So Sir Thomas reluctantly agreed. "So be it, I shall call them off. Terror, Dare come." Sir Thomas' request was denied. None of the dogs stopped barking. Sir Thomas shook his head with a quick movement, surprised. "I do not understand. Dare has never disobeyed me like this before." So he tried again. "Terror, Dare, stop!" Again Dare, along with all the dogs, ignored this command.

Lord Riley and Sherman III became even more terrified. Both begged for their lives. "Pray, Sir Thomas, make them stop! Call them off!" When they looked into the dogs' eyes, both could tell, especially Lord Riley, that these dogs knew the evil that lurked within their hearts. The dogs knew that a lot of innocent blood had been shed because of these two evil men, and that much more would be shed unless they were stopped.

Lord Riley demanded and threatened, "Take charge, Sir Thomas! Be firm with your beast, lest he and his pack kill us, in which case you shall be charged with murder!"

Sir Thomas ignorantly took Lord Riley's advice. He yelled, "Dare, stop! I command thee!" Dare turned and looked at his master. He was growling and foaming at the mouth, with his fangs completely exposed. This even sent chills up Sir Thomas' spine. He took two steps backwards mumbling, "'Tis not my dog." He paused a second in disbelief before continuing, "I do fear that a Hellhound spirit from the forest hath taken over." Dare turned side ways, barking into Terror's ear. Terror barked back, and turned around and faced Sir Thomas with a crazed, starved expression. Sir Thomas trembled with fear from this expression. He raised both hands as Terror crept towards him, hunched over. "Good dog Terror! Good dog!" Sir Thomas continually said as he slowly walked backwards.

Seeing this, Sherman III and Lord Riley continued to beg, "Do not forsake us, Sir Thomas! Stay and command them to stop."

Sir Thomas replied as he kept slowly stepping backwards. "You command Terror to stop. He once belonged to you." The dogs were now in a circle around Lord Riley and Sherman III right in front of their faces. Both men could feel saliva from the dogs pour on them as the dogs continued to bark furiously. In the past, Lord Riley had been very successful at making his dogs enraged, but he never saw dogs half this enraged before. Now petrified, Lord Riley felt like these dogs were judges reading his soul, and were moments away from sentencing him to a long, painful death. Knowing that Sherman III and Lord Riley's life was in danger, Sir Thomas stopped backing up, ignoring Terror's snarls and looks of kill. He screamed at the pack, "NO!" as Terror lunged and grabbed the back of Sir Thomas' collar with his teeth and dragged him away from there on his back. Sir Thomas, in fear for his life, attempted to scream, "Help Dare!" but could only mumble these words because he was being choked by being dragged. Dare ignored his master's plea, for he was completely focused on Lord Riley and Sherman III.

While Sir Thomas was being dragged away, Lord Riley and Sherman III again pleaded with Dare for their lives. "We implore you to let us live. We are sorry for what we did to Sir Thomas' uncle. If you let us live, we promise we will never hurt any one close to your master again."

*Dare made his thoughts aware with a glare,*
*as Lord Riley and Sherman III stared scared.*
*"Enough with the lying eyes! I see through your disguise,*
*through the gateway of your soul, I see thoughts unthinkable*
*giving me a rage unquenchable, so woe to you foe, for your crime is*
*unforgivable, the terrible disaster, of taking the uncle's life of my beloved*
*master, you bloody bastard, it's now your sorry ass I am after; soon you will*
*not feel well, in fact you'll holler and yell, with pain so insane, due to blood*
*gushing out your membrane, you've brought great sorrow, for you there is no*
*tomorrow, for when my mouth is full, I shall crush your skull."*

These words went through Sherman III and Lord Riley's minds during the brief moments that they stared in Dare's eyes.

Sir Thomas, by now having been dragged five hundred feet away on his back, was rolled over on his stomach. Terror stood over him, growling as he placed his jaws over the back of Sir Thomas neck, keeping him pinned. Sir Thomas intelligently lay still as a board, knowing it would take these powerful jaws no more than three seconds to crush and end his life. In a calm, quiet voice, Sir Thomas chanted over and over.

*"In Jesus name I pray, Hellhound spirit go away!"*
*These words were to of no avail. Terror even wiggled his tail,*
*finding this chant amusingly frail.*

A few seconds later, Terror lifted his head straight up releasing a loud howl. When done, he continued growling, placing his jaws back around Sir Thomas' neck. Sherman III, hearing Terror's loud howl, figured that this was the signal for the dogs to begin attacking. Therefore, with the sword in his left hand, he attempted to slice the giant dog across the throat. Dare's sister leaped, preventing this by biting the right side of his face. Her big front tooth made contact with his eyeball, crushing half of it out. Sherman III screamed in agony, managing somehow to hold onto his swords. Now, the sword in his left hand came across his body towards Dare's sister's throat, instead of going towards the giant dog, No pain was too great to restrain him back from attacking her. However, one of her beloved sons leaped with precise timing for Sherman III left wrist, and crushed it in multiple places with his bites. The sword of Sherman III flew out of his hand a couple of inches away from Dare's sister's throat. The whole side of the sword bounced harmlessly off of her back, as the pack commenced to attack, knocking Lord Riley and Sherman III to the ground crushing bones and ripping flesh. Lord Riley now joined his cousin, screaming in agony, as Dare's sister stood shoulder to shoulder next to her brother as they savagely attacked Lord Riley. The dogs over the next three hours slowly munched away, eating Lord Riley and Sherman III alive. The dogs ate every part of their bodies, starting with the fingers and toes, and leaving the heads for last. When done, all dogs lay full next to one another. Dare burped, afterwards lifted his head in the air howling. His master was still pinned to the ground with imprints of fangs pressed against the back of his neck. Hearing Dare's howl, Terror released Sir Thomas who rolled over on his back staring up in the sky still petrified. Terror began to lick Sir Thomas' face and neck while wagging his tail.

Sir Thomas's hands were shaking as he slowly and gently petted Terror's head, while he looked toward the sky, "Thank you, Jesus, for answering my prayer, freeing Terror from the evil Hellhound spirit which so powerfully dwelt in him." Sir Thomas, after taking a saliva bath from Terror (over the next few minutes) calmed down and rose to his feet. They walked back to Dare and the rest of the dogs, who were all lying, down licking one another's lips. Sir Thomas noticed before Terror pinned him that every single dog there had thin stomach's, with most of their ribs showing. Now all the dog's stomachs were fat, with none of their ribs showing. Sir Thomas walked over to Dare, dazed and confused. Dare wagged his tail along with his whole body. He was happy to see his master and to know that his master's life, along with countless numbers of dog's lives, would no longer be in danger from Lord Riley and Sherman III. Sir Thomas petted Dare on the top of his head. "What went on over here while I was gone? Where are Lord Riley and Vivian's father? There is no sign of them any where." Sir Thomas looked in the midst of the dogs and saw Sherman III's swords lying there. "That is rather odd," he said, confused, "I wonder why Vivian's father did not take his swords with him." Just then Sir Thomas heard a few of the dogs release long, loud, absurd farts. "Ahhh! If thou must fart, hath heart, warn before tis blown apart." Sir Thomas said as he cringed gasping, flapping his hand across his face, trying to avoid smelling the stench. At that moment, a gory thought popped in his head. *Is it possible that Dare and these dogs ate Lord Riley and Sherman III?* After a couple of seconds of pondering on this thought, Sir Thomas waved his hand down, shaking his head, "No

- what a ludicrous thought." Then he turned towards Dare's sister, petting her on the head while giving her a big hug as she happily wiggled her tail. "Thou must be me dog's sister." I can see the strong resemblance. Our thanks for saving us. We owe you our lives." Dare's sister responded by licking him in the face while farting. Sir Thomas smiled, rising to his feet. He walked by all the dogs, petting, hugging thanking each, as Dare walked by all the dogs licking their lips. When Sir Thomas addressed Terror, he dropped to his knees with a tear, giving him the biggest hug of all, "Well my friend," Sir Thomas sadly said, "Dare and I are really going to miss thee. Both of us are delighted to know that you now have a wonderful family and are going to be alright." Afterwards Sir Thomas rose to his feet, wiped the tear from his eye and started heading home. He took ten steps when a mouth gently nipped at his ankle. Sir Thomas stopped, and turned around. Terror sat looking up at him with his head tilted sideways. Terror wasn't done saying goodbye. He wiggled his tail, stretching out his paw and shaking Sir Thomas's hand with a sad but happy look, telling him with his eyes, "Thanks for resurrecting my spirit with your kind, powerful love. I shall always remember and love you." Sir Thomas shed a few happy and sad tears as he wrapped his arms back around Terror. After saying a long goodbye, Sir Thomas rose to his feet drying his eyes, saying, "I would really love to stay longer, but Dare and I really have to get home." Dare, overly full, followed his master, wiggling his tail, walking as slow as a snail.

On their way home, Sir Thomas tried to make Dare walk faster by saying, "Come on Dare, hurry up! What's wrong, thou mad beast? I have never seen thee move so slowly in your life! Mother and father are probably worried sick about us!" (Sir Thomas had no idea how worried.) Sir Thomas and Dare hiked all through the day and deep into the night, eventually showing up at home. At the time, Sir Thomas' parents were cuddled up next to the fire, praying for their son to come home safe and soon.

When they heard the door knock, both of them jumped to their feet, running towards the door. "Is that my son?" asked his mother.

"Yes mother, 'tis I." Sir Thomas answered, tired. "Dare and I are home now." The door swung open. Both parents embraced their son, crying tears of joy while looking up and thanking God, and petting Dare who happily wiggled his tail.

Sir Thomas' mother stared into her son's eyes. "Are ye two alright?" she asked, concerned.

With eyes half closed from being tired, Sir Thomas nodded. "Yes mother, but we are, both very hungry, especially Dare. You should have seen how slowly he walked home! I think he may have lost strength from not eating."

Mrs. Gentry jumped to her feet and ran into the kitchen, bringing out some bread for her son and raw meat for Dare. Sir Thomas quickly ate the bread. "Thanks mother, that was the best tasting bread, I have ever eaten in my life." Sir Thomas, deeply concerned, turned to his parents with a serious look asking, "How is Uncle Robert?" Mr. Gentry quickly ran out of the room crying, as Mrs. Gentry hugged her son with tears in her eyes.

"I am so sorry son. Your uncle was murdered the day before yesterday."

Sir Thomas hearing this instantly bawled like a baby, screaming "NO! NO! You bloody bastard Lord Riley! You shall burn in hell!"

Mrs. Gentry nodded her head, agreeing that it was Lord Riley. With deep concern she responded, "We feel that your life is in great danger from him and his cousin Sherman III. The authorities are searching to interrogate them, but haven't a clue where they are."

*Sir Thomas abruptly turned his head towards Dare.*
*Who lay sideways on the floor, his stomach fuller then a boar,*
*for the first time in Dare's life he refused to eat fresh, raw meat.*
*Forcing himself to his feet, with a pain in his heart,*
*he soon released a loud stench fart,*
*walking and barking he headed for the door,*
*his stomach in a gassy uproar, Sir Thomas quickly rose, plugged his nose,*
*as he opened the door. No more steps were taken than four,*
*when out squirted Lord Riley, which Dare avoided, crapping on the floor.*

Sir Thomas noticed a strange familiar stench coming from the diarrhea. He walked over to look at it. In the bright light of the full moon, he was able to clearly see, which put his mind a little at ease, for mixed in the diarrhea were little bits and pieces of crushed bone and a shirt resembling the one Lord Riley had worn. Sir Thomas knew then and there why he had been dragged by Terror and pinned to the ground for so long. Dare knew that Lord Riley and Sherman III had killed his uncle and had absolutely no remorse for doing so. Dare wanted his wicked foes to know just how much Robert was loved, and to feel the wrath of the Gentry family, by torturing them to a slow horrifying death. Sir Thomas knew this was a bloody massacre, one which would have planted a morbid imprint in his mind for a very long time to come. Sir Thomas hugged Dare while looking up at his mother.

*"Ask me no questions, I'll tell you no lies,*
*Sherman III and Lord Riley will not be found to give any alibis!"*

And so it was that fight number two between Terror and Brahma the Bull was cancelled. Bull bating took a big step backwards and church attendance quickly grew. However, eight weeks after the death of Lord Riley and Sherman III, Emerald gave birth to a nice healthy litter of nine. Vivian was there and was ecstatic about the litter. He picked up one of the two biggest puppies, which had markings just like Terror and carried him over to a giant bull in a barn. Holding the pup up to the bulls face Vivian said, "BEHOLD, THY WORST NIGHTMARE!"

www.ingramcontent.com/pod-product-compliance
Lightning Source LLC
Chambersburg PA
CBHW031926190326
41519CB00007B/427